THE COMPLETE GUIDE TO

AEROBIC DANCING

BY BETH A. KUNTZLEMAN AND THE EDITORS OF CONSUMER GUIDE®

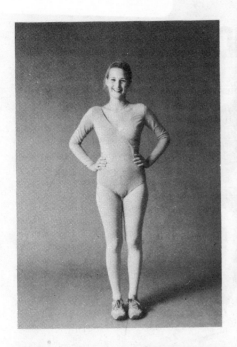
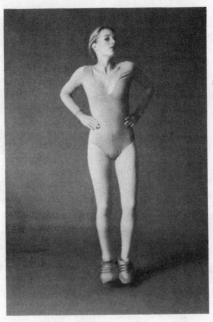
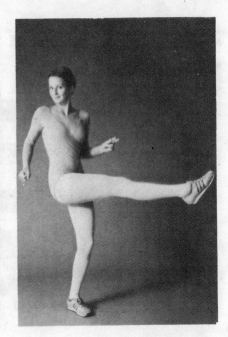

Contents

IMPORTANT! READ THE FIRST FOUR CHAPTERS BEFORE BEGINNING THE PROGRAM!

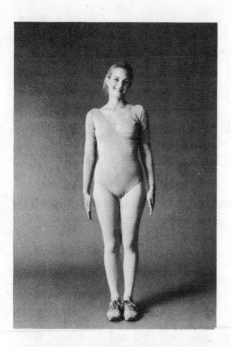
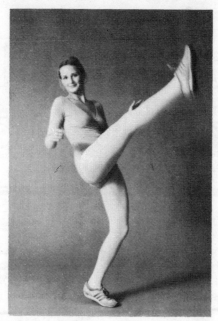
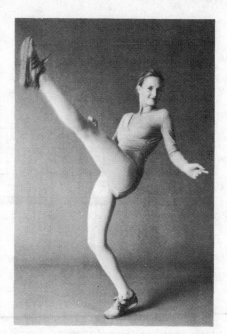

The Routines (continued)

When you've learned all our routines, you'll be ready to go it alone.

Publisher
Louis Weber

Editor-In-Chief
Jerold L. Kellman

Managing Editor
Greg Erickson

Editors
Bob Schmidt
Carole Turko
Chris Poole

Special Projects Editors
Geraldine Lynch
Tobi Kelmer

Production Director
Geraldine Lynch

Assistant Production Manager
Debby Davis Eisel

Production Editors
Debra Sostrin
Bonnie M. Cassidy
Helen Clark

.Editorial Assistants
Gloria Goldberg
Amy Okrei
Gert Salzenstein
Marla Kaye
Jeryl Minow

Art Director
Frank E. Peiler

Art Department Manager
Brenda Kaharl

Art Assistants
Mary Jo Roche
Quan Lee
Sharon Schroeder

President
Louis Weber

Executive Vice-President
Estelle Weber

Vice-Presidents
Frank E. Peiler
Jack Lynn

Marketing Director
Steven Feinberg

Circulation Manager
Edward Geraghty

Cover Design
Frank E. Peiler

Photographs
Kurt Brabbèe

Editorial & Subscription Offices: 3841 W. Oakton Street, Skokie, IL 60076

CONSUMER GUIDE® magazine Health Quarterly Winter 1980. Volume 253

CONSUMER GUIDE® magazine Health Quarterly is published 4 times a year.

Why Are All These People Dancing?

Every aerobic dancer seems to have a different reason for taking up the program. Some benefits of aerobic dance can be measured—with a bathroom scale, a tape measure, or a blood pressure gauge. Others are less tangible. People dance because it makes them feel better or more sexy or energetic. Many people get into aerobic dance simply because it's fun.

Let's take a look at the benefits you can expect from your aerobic dance program.

Weight Control

Physical activity is the key to weight control. Studies have shown that the non-obese person often eats as much as the obese. Dr. Jean Mayer, Ph.D, former professor of nutrition at Harvard University, worked with overweight high school girls. His results indicated that they ate no more, and some ate less, than their classmates of normal weight. But, the overweight girls exercised far less and went in for more "sitting" activities than did the thinner girls. In fact, they spent a considerably greater amount of time watching TV than did the others. And, during their active periods, they chose to stand more frequently than the non-obese. Similar studies done with boys and adults have come to the same conclusion. Fat accumulates not so much because of overeating, but because of underdoing.

The most cogent statement regarding weight control and activity has been made by the world-famous Mayer. "I'm convinced that inactivity is the most important factor explaining the frequency of 'creeping overweight' in modern society. Our body's regulation of food intake was just not designed for the highly-mechanized condition of modern life . . . adapting to these conditions without developing obesity means either that the individual will have to step up his activity or he will be mildly or acutely hungry all of his life."[1]

Your body maintains a fine balance between the number of calories you eat and the number of calories you burn off through physical activity. If you take in more calories than you burn off, you will gain weight. The extra calories will be stored as fat in your body.

The reverse is also true. If you eat fewer calories than you burn off, you will lose weight. Your body will call on its fat cells to release fat for energy.

Skeptics point out that it takes a great deal of exercise to burn off the calorie equivalent of one pound of fat. It is true that 10 minutes of high-intensity aerobic dancing will use up only 100 calories, or 1/35th of a pound. That doesn't sound like much perhaps. But, exercise, like eating, has a cumulative effect. If you dance 30 minutes a day, six days a week, you'll lose a pound every two weeks, or around 25 pounds a year.

Dr. Herbert Weber, Ph.D., professor of physical education at East Stroudsburg State College, conducted a study on a group of 10 aerobic dancers who ranged in skill from novice to advanced. The average age of the women was 35; their average weight, 117. Each woman performed her dancing routine with a portable respirometer on her back. This piece of equipment resembles scuba-diving gear. It measures the number of calories burned.

The women did low-, moderate-, and high-intensity dance workouts. Weber's study showed that women working at a low level of aerobic dance used about four calories per minute. At the moderate level they used about six calories per minute. And at the high level they used about nine calories per minute.

Calories Used Per Hour of Aerobic Dancing

Intensity of Workout	Body Weight In Pounds						
	100	120	140	150	160	180	200
Low	215	230	245	260	275	290	305
Moderate	350	375	395	420	445	470	490
High	515	550	585	620	655	690	725

That means low-intensity aerobic dance is the equivalent of such activities as archery, golf, horseshoe pitching, and walking two-and-a-half miles per hour. Moderate-intensity dance is equivalent to ice skating at nine miles per hour, walking at three-and-a-half miles per hour, or bicycling at about 10 miles per hour. High-intensity aerobic dance is similar to vigorous basketball, social handball, bicycling at 13 miles per hour, fencing, playing squash, and running or jogging at five-and-a-half to six miles per hour.

Dr. Weber's conclusion on aerobic dance and weight control is clear: "If pursued regularly with adequate intensity, the dance's caloric cost could complement a sensible diet for purposes of weight control."[2]

Fat Loss

When people lose weight by dieting they often complain that they still look flabby. And they do. That is because they lose fat *and* lean body tissues. Fat is fat, but lean body tissue is what makes up the muscles and organs of your body. Lean body tissue gives you your shape. Proper exercise results in weight loss and in fat loss, but without loss in lean body tissue.

Drs. Bill Zuti, Ph.D., and Lawrence Golding, Ph.D., conducted a study that illustrates this point. They set out to compare the effects of several different methods of weight reduction. The 25 women participating in the study were all between the ages of 25 and 40, and were 20 to 40 pounds overweight. Three groups were formed: (1) eight women went on a diet, reducing their caloric intake by 500 calories per day, but holding their physical activity constant; (2) nine continued to eat as usual, but increased physical activity to burn off 500 extra calories a day; and (3) eight reduced caloric intake by 250 calories a day and increased physical activity to burn off 250 extra calories per day. Before and after the 16-week period, the subjects were tested for body weight, body density, skin-fold and girth measurements, and selected blood lipids (fats).

The results indicated that there was no significant difference between the groups in the amount of weight lost. The average individual weight loss in all three groups was 11.4 pounds. But there was a difference between the groups with regard to body composition. Those in the exercise group and in the combination exercise/diet group had undergone significant changes in body density. The dieting group lost both body fat and muscle tissue; the exercise groups lost more body fat and no muscle tissue.

The members of the exercise groups reaped other benefits too: they had more stamina than the others and their circulatory systems were better able to withstand the rigors of exercise. The report concluded that the use of exercise in a weight-reduction program is far superior to dieting alone in its effect on body composition and physical fitness.[3]

Cardiovascular Fitness

Your body needs oxygen to keep going. You can deprive yourself of food for a few weeks, or water for several days. But try holding your breath for more than a few minutes, and see what happens. Oxygen is vital if you want to stay alive. Oxygen passes from the lungs into every cell of your body. It travels through a series of blood vessels, and it's moved by a very important pump, your heart. The heart is an incredibly efficient organ that works night and day with no rest (other than the split second between beats). The human heart usually beats between 60 and 80 times a minute. With each beat, it pumps about 130 cubic centimeters of blood or five liters (a little over five quarts) of blood each minute. In your lifetime of 70 years it may beat two-and-a-half billion times.

You must care for your heart to keep it working at optimum efficiency. One of the things you can do to take care of your heart is to get regular, proper exercise. Aerobic exercises keep your heart healthy and increase the body's ability to use oxygen. Dancing, swimming, rowing, walking, running, and bicycling—any exercise or sport, in fact, that requires a sustained activity over a long period—are aerobic exercises.

Aerobic exercise teaches your body to be more efficient. Your heart will pump the same amount of blood with fewer beats. Countless studies have shown that while the heart of the average sedentary person beats about 60 to 80 times each minute at rest, the heart of the aerobic exerciser generally beats only 40 to 50 times each minute. And, although it's beating at about half the average rate, the aerobically-conditioned heart circulates the same amount of oxygen-rich blood throughout the body. How can this happen when the heart is only working at half power?

The truth is that the heart conditioned by aerobic exercise beats more strongly and deeply. That is, with each beat the conditioned heart pumps more blood. The aerobic exerciser's conditioned heart, working at half the average rate, gets more rest between beats and will probably last longer. And not only the heart benefits from aerobic exercise. The lungs of the aerobic exerciser also become more highly conditioned. When well conditioned, they'll take in more oxygen.

Aerobic dance produces the same benefits as other types of aerobic training. It improves cardiovascular fitness. Sonia Maas at North Texas State University studied 31 women who performed aerobic dance routines 30 to 40 minutes each day for 12 weeks. At the conclusion of the study the women had lowered their resting heart rates, improved their ability to tolerate high exercise loads, and improved their performance on a 12-minute run/walk test—a gauge of aerobic capacity.[4]

Dr. Weber, in the study previously cited, noted that investigators could "observe that high-intensity aerobic dancing was physically taxing. The heavy sweating, breathlessness, and fatigue made it impossible to differentiate our dancers from other exercisers competing in a half hour of basketball, handball, jogging, and the like."[5] Sophisticated testing supported their observations. The data showed that if approached moderately or vigorously aerobic dance could produce enough metabolic or cardiovascular stress to develop physical fitness.

Aerobic dance is a bona fide aerobic exercise. It improves your cardiovascular fitness. Your heart will pump more blood with fewer beats. Your body will be able to pick up, transport, and use oxygen more efficiently. Your muscles will get stronger and more efficient. You will "get into shape." You'll have more energy and you'll be less tired.

Proper exercise will also reduce your chance of developing heart disease. Recent studies have shown that active people are less prone to heart disease than are the sedentary. Dr. Kenneth Cooper, M.D., for example, conducted a study in which he compared a person's level of aerobic capacity, or fitness level, with selected heart-disease risk factors. The study indicated that as a person's fitness level improves, his risk of getting heart-disease drops substantially. The study showed a straight-line relationship between physical activity and the reduction of risk factors. People in very poor or poor aerobic fitness ran a greater risk of getting heart disease than did those in fair aerobic fitness. And those in the good or excellent fitness category had the lowest scores on selected heart disease risk factors.

Perhaps all these studies are best summarized by Drs. Samuel Fox, M.D., and William Haskell, Ph.D.: "There is not enough evidence to prove that exercise prevents heart disease, but it certainly is considered by many to be a promising field of investigation and a prudent practice for most people to follow."[6]

Of course, doing aerobic exercise is not an absolute guarantee that you won't get heart disease, but it does seem to provide some pretty good health insurance.

Body Toning and Appearance

Aerobic dance will do wonders for your body. Improved body tone is one of its most noticeable benefits. A well-toned body is one in which all muscles are firm, well-shaped, and visually appealing.

Aerobic dance can also help you achieve better body posture and carriage. Have you ever watched people walk? Some of them slump, some of them slide, some of them send their stomachs first. Some totter, some waddle, some plod, and some march like toy soldiers.

Other people walk with a posture and bearing that says: Here is somebody special. This somebody special doesn't have to be a very big person, or beautiful, or handsome, or well-dressed. No, these people stand out in a crowd because of the way they carry themselves. Their posture breathes self-confidence, composure, and grace.

Good carriage does not come naturally. We have to work to attain it. You have to train the muscles that enable you to stand, walk, and sit properly. And, once you've trained yourself to move smoothly and properly, you place less strain on the back muscles, have fewer back problems, and suffer less fatigue. In short, improving your carriage and posture will increase your overall vitality—one of the many benefits derived from a well-balanced body. Aerobic dance can give you this good carriage and posture.

Another distinct physical benefit of an aerobic dance program is the slowing and possible improvement of varicose veins. Obese people and pregnant women are especially susceptible to varicose veins in the legs. Excess abdominal weight exerts pressure on the large veins in the legs. This pressure, in turn, restricts blood flow and causes the valves in the veins to function improperly. Blood can pool and push the veins toward the body surface, causing the unsightly condition we call varicose veins.

A well-rounded aerobic dance program will strengthen the abdomen and prevent this pressure from being exerted on leg veins. The various dance steps and exercises that concentrate on the legs will massage these veins and help them regain, or retain, their elasticity, thus helping to keep these veins in their proper place.

General Well-Being

Most aerobic dancers start their program with the aims of trimming their bodies and losing weight. And, as we have seen, these goals can be accomplished through a regular program of aerobic dance. Why, then, do they stick with the program after they've slimmed down and firmed up? Most stick with it because it provides a psychological lift. It's as though the exercise were a "tune-up" for the mind.

Aerobic dance, you see, will clear the mental cobwebs that have been hanging around inside your head for so long. Most dancers say they start to feel their capacities picking up in all areas of their life as they begin to feel better physically. That doesn't mean you'll be transformed into a genius simply by dancing a few minutes each week, but dancing may help reduce energy-robbing tensions and depression that block your imaginative thinking.

Most of us suffer from ordinary psychological blahs caused by the garden-variety tensions and stresses common in modern life. Many people complain of mysterious aches and pains, depression, and lack of energy. They're often not up to any entertainment or recreation other than an evening with the "tube."

Research has shown that proper aerobic exercise is an effective antidote for these ills. It combats tension, reduces fatigue, and increases energy. By providing you with a sense of accomplishment, it improves your self-image. Over a generation ago the late Dr. Paul Dudley White, M.D., dean of American cardiologists, said: "Vigorous leg exercise is the best antidote for nervous and emotional stress that we possess, far better than tranquilizers or sedatives to which, unhappily, so many are addicted today."[7]

Recent research supports his contention. Dr. Herbert deVries, Ph.D., working with a group of men 50 years old and older, discovered that a 15-minute walk reduced neuromuscular tension more effectively than did a dose of tranquilizers.[8]

Dr. Herbert Weber after investigating the effects of aerobic dancing on the body noted that aerobic dancing "promotes positive feelings of well-being . . . it's an activity that offers sufficient variety and creative opportunities to sustain the participants' interest and prevent them from becoming exercise 'dropouts'."[9]

How can aerobic dance do this?

For an answer, let's listen to these aerobic dance experts: Jacki Sorensen, the founder of aerobic dancing in America, notes that "aerobic dancing is fun! Dances are choreographed to be simple enough for the 'non-dancing man,' woman, or child, yet challenging enough not to be boring. Those participating in an aerobic dancing program are encouraged to have FUN moving by doing the routines with their own special style, and within their individual limits of coordination, reaction time, flexibility, and endurance . . . the goal is fun and fitness, not perfection of specific skills."[10]

Lynnette Handley, developer of Dancefit and consultant for the Detroit YMCA, says aerobic dance exercise "combines the basic elements of a good fitness workout with the fun of dancing . . .

adding the pure joy of dancing, not for technique but for the fun of it . . . makes us forget that we are really exercising. Music is a source of pure amazement when we realize how it can change our moods and make us want to move."[11]

Participation in aerobic dance gives you a feeling of accomplishment. Aerobic dancers learn, often dramatically, that they can change themselves for the better. They see that they can control their lives to improve their health, appearance, and self-image.

Getting your body into shape makes you feel good. We all know what happens when we don't exercise. Those nearly perfect, youthful bodies begin to develop fat places and skinny places, sags and bulges. We stop growing at both ends, but we often continue to grow in our middles, especially if we have sit-down-behind-the-desk jobs. Some people develop pot bellies; others hunch and stoop, especially if they are tall. Women find themselves with less-than-firm busts and feel generally flabby. Result? Our self-esteem falters. Our self-image suffers. We get "down on ourselves." Good physical exercise can reverse all this.

When you start to look good again, you start to feel better about yourself. With a regular routine of aerobic dance, your body—that tremendously complex and responsive natural machine that you were born with—will regain its tone. People who have participated in aerobic dance for a few weeks feel great because they look good. Feeling good about yourself can bring more joy into your life.

Finally, proper aerobic exercise will give you more energy. With physical conditioning comes a greater capacity to get things done. You will be able to do more before feeling tired. You will have more pep.

Aerobic dancing is not a panacea for your aches, pains, and ailments—whether physical or mental. But it can make a large contribution to your physical and mental well-being. A regular program of aerobic dance can make you look and feel better. It will make you proud of your body. It will give you stamina and better health. It's a super package deal—better health, appearance, and feelings.

[1] Jean Mayer, *Overweight: Causes, Cost, and Control.* (Englewood Cliffs, NJ: Prentice-Hall, 1968), p. 82.

[2] H. Weber, "The Energy Cost of Aerobic Dance." *Fitness For Living*, Volume 8, No. 2, (March/April, 1974), p. 30.

[3] B. Zuti and L. Golding, "Comparing Diet and Exercise As Weight Reduction Tools," *The Physician and Sportsmedicine*, January, 1976: p. 49.

[4] Maas, Sonia H., "A Study Of The Cardiovascular Training Effects Of Aerobic Dance Instruction Among College-Age Females," (Master's Thesis, North Texas State University, 1975).

[5] Weber, "The Energy Cost of Aerobic Dancing," p. 26.

[6] S.M. Fox and W.L. Haskell, "Population Studies," *Canadian Medical Association Journal*, 96:1967: pp. 806-810.

[7] P.D. White, "Health," in C.T. Kuntzleman (ed.), *The Physical Fitness Encyclopedia.* (Emmaus, PA: Rodale Press, 1970), pp. 214-215.

[8] H.A. deVries and G.M. Adams, "Electromyographic Comparison of Single Doses of Exercise and Meprobamate as to the Effects on Muscular Relaxation," *American Journal of Physical Medicine*, 51:1972: pp. 130-141.

[9] Weber, "The Energy Cost of Aerobic Dancing," p. 30.

[10] J. Sorensen, "Aerobic Dancing." President's Council on Physical Fitness and Sports, n.d., p. 2.

[11] Lynnette Handley. *DanceFIT*, n.d., p. 2.

Getting Started

Right now you may want to turn on the music and start hopping and high-stepping your way to fitness. But a word of caution is in order. For the sake of your health, and to reduce the chance of injury, be sensible. Proceed slowly at first, especially if the most exercise you've had in the last year has been getting up and down to switch channels.

See Your Doctor First

If you have any questions about your health, check with your doctor. Of course, we also recommend that those who choose to be sedentary see their doctor. After all, it's been shown that inactive people are far more likely to suffer from obesity, heart disease, back problems, and other ailments than are those who exercise. Choosing to be sedentary is a risky decision.

A few people have a condition that precludes participation in aerobic exercise. Some diseases, such as advanced arthritis, diabetes, consistent pains of the lower back, orthopedic problems, and various conditions of the liver and kidneys, may make aerobic dance impossible and painful.

Even if you feel confident that you don't have any of these ailments, you would be well advised to have a general checkup. It's possible to have one of these diseases without knowing it. Some other medical factor may also rule out aerobic dance for you. Use common sense. Talk things over with your doctor. State what you plan to do, have an examination, ask for advice, and follow it. It would be a good idea to bring this book along and discuss its contents.

Once in the doctor's office, make certain an electrocardiogram (ECG) is included in the examination, especially if you're past the age of 35. One of the most important tests that can be given for exercisers, the ECG evaluates the performance of the heart and reveals abnormalities that might force you to abandon or modify your aerobic dance program.

Two kinds of ECG examinations are generally available to test your heart: the resting ECG and the stress ECG (also called stress test). The resting ECG tests your heart while you're lying down. Consequently, it does not show how your heart performs when it is working under stress or exercise conditions.

Through the stress test the doctor tries to find out what happens to your body when you're exercising. In a stress test you walk or run on a treadmill or ride a bicycle at progressively faster speeds or against increasing resistance. As the exercise load steadily increases, the stress on your heart also increases. Consequently, your heart beats faster and faster. Electronic devices record your heartbeat and monitor your heart's key functions until your heart rate gets to at least 75 percent of your maximum rate. (Your maximum heart rate and the method of determining it for yourself are discussed in the CONSUMER GUIDE® Aerobic Dancing Program chapter.) Some doctors will permit you to exercise to your maximum. If your heart starts to show some abnormal changes before you reach the desired cutoff point, your test may be terminated sooner.

Not all doctors are equipped to conduct a stress test in their office. But they can send you to a hospital which has the necessary facilities for conducting the test.

Although a stress ECG costs about $100 to $150, it is worthwhile if you can afford it. In any case, an ordinary medical checkup which includes a resting ECG is important if you're getting past the age of 35.

Getting Ready

Your body needs a period of preconditioning before you can get into real training. In our aerobic dance program, learning the routines serves as preconditioning. These exercises help your muscles, heart, and lungs adjust to the increased exercise load.

Your preconditioning program will be speeded up if you learn to incorporate walking into your life. Leave your car behind if you're not going very far. Walk to the store, walk to the movies, visit a friend with your feet instead of your car. Try to break the habit of reaching for your car keys. Stop the urge to drive every place you have to go.

If it's convenient, walk to work. If not, park your car farther from the office or train station than is usual and walk the rest of the way. Stay away from escalators and elevators; use the stairs. If your office is on the eighteenth floor, take the stairs part of the way and make the rest of the trip in the elevator. Make a brisk 10-to-15 minute walk after dinner a regular part of your evening. If you get into habits like these, it won't be long before your body will tell you that you are ready for aerobic dance.

When To Dance

It's important to establish your own routine, geared to your disposition and living habits. Some people like to dance early in the morning, others at midday and others at night. If you're a morning person and like to get up with the larks, aerobic dance in the morning would be a great wake-up routine. If you're the sort who spends most of the morning groping around trying to get your eyes open, don't force yourself to greet the dawn. Leave it to the larks. Dance later in the day when it fits your metabolism and idiosyncrasies.

Once you have decided on the best time for you to dance, stick to it. If one day you dance in the morning, and the next day in the mid-afternoon, and the third in the evening, you're not building a strong routine. Strive to develop a new habit of exercise, a habit you will keep up for the rest of your life. This is much easier to do if you exercise at the same time every day.

When Not To Dance

Recommended schedules should be followed as faithfully as possible, but not blindly. There are certain times when you have no business dancing. If, for example, you have the flu, a cold, or some other ailment, don't overexert yourself by trying to dance. If you feel a cold coming on, it's best to lay low.

And don't dance when you've been drinking. Although some people say that vigorous exercising is a great way to overcome a hangover, it's just not worth the possibility that you'll hurt yourself. To compound the problem, some of the routines we're going to ask you to do may be difficult if you're a little tipsy or not feeling up to par.

Where To Do It

Thousands of people these days go to the "Y" or a local health club to do their aerobic dancing. However, there are several real advantages in aerobic dance at home:
1. You do not have to adjust your schedule to that of a large institution.

2. You don't have to spend the time traveling.
3. You can perform your aerobic dancing routines without feeling self-conscious.

Where in the house though? You'll need enough space to move around. Check out your home, room by room, corner to corner. A room 20 by 15 feet is sufficient, but you may have to be content with a smaller area.

If your house or apartment has large rooms, space will probably not be a problem. If you live in a small house or apartment, however, you may want to consider moving the furniture so that you can dance. And, when choosing your dance site, make sure the ceiling is high enough to permit you to extend your arms fully overhead. If you live on the second or third floor, you must consider the feelings of the person below you. You may have to dance when your neighbor is out of the house, or perhaps you could convince the landlord to let you use the garage or basement.

Make sure your exercise space is well ventilated, and try to keep the temperature relatively cool—60° to 65°F.—but avoid cold air from air conditioning or an open window.

Set a Goal

Goals give you something specific to work toward. They provide a standard by which to measure your progress. When you set a goal, avoid generalizations such as "I want to get into shape," or "I want to lose weight." Instead, set a specific long-term goal and some short-term goals.

For example, if you want to lose weight, decide what your best weight would be and give yourself six months or a year to reach that weight. Set a short-term goal of losing three pounds by the end of the first month. Achieving your short-term goal will give you the motivation to reach that long-term goal.

What To Wear

Wear whatever is comfortable when you dance. Leotards, tights, shorts and T-shirt, or a light exercise suit—anything that will allow your body to move and breathe freely—would be fine.

However, there is one essential: good running shoes. All the hopping, skipping, jumping, running in place, and dance steps can be traumatic to your feet and legs. A good running shoe can help your feet and legs absorb the blows.

The selection of a good running shoe is not simple. You want to be certain that the shoe provides good support and cups the heel. It should also have firm arch support, good protection at the ball of the foot, and a flexible front sole. A good pair of shoes will make your dancing more comfortable and will help prevent injuries and ailments.

The CONSUMER GUIDE® Aerobic Dancing Program

Your heart and respiratory systems are the power plants that drive your body. They might be better described as two interdependent systems in a single power plant. In simplest terms, the lungs take in the oxygen the body needs to "burn" food, which is your body's fuel. Waste gases are given off in the form of carbon dioxide. A transport system carries the oxygen from the lungs to the cells and then carries off the waste carbon dioxide to be exhaled. The blood vessels and the heart provide the transport system—a complicated arrangement of pipes and a simple yet extraordinary pump. If the lungs take in less oxygen than is needed, the body cells are deprived of oxygen. If the heart and blood cannot transport oxygen as fast as the lungs can take it in, the same deprivation occurs. Obviously, if both systems are crippled, the body's cells suffer even more.

Any worthwhile physical fitness program must focus on these two systems and their mutual dependence. According to the American Heart Association's Committee on Exercise and Fitness and the American College of Sports Medicine, an exercise contributes to cardiovascular fitness only if it involves both systems and is sustained for at least 15 minutes, and preferably 20 minutes or more. That is why a game of tennis, even a spirited one, is not the most useful exercise to strengthen the heart and lungs. A typical tennis game has periods of furious activity, full of lunging and running and rapid stops and starts. But these active periods are too short, and there is too much rest in between. The action is not sustained.

Our aerobic dance program is based on the principle of continuous action. It is designed to keep you moving. If at any time you forget a step or must wait for a record to change, you simply keep your legs in motion until you fall back into the mainstream of things.

The program is structured to enable you to proceed at your own pace through successive stages according to your personal timetable. When you're ready to move ahead, you do. If you're not ready to go to a higher level of conditioning, you wait until you are.

Your Maximum Heart Rate

Everyone has what is called a "maximum heart rate"—generally based on age and current physical condition. A person's maximum heart rate is the number of times the heart beats per minute when the body is undergoing maximum exertion. The maximum heart rate is generally figured to be

220 beats per minute minus your age. If you're 20 years old, your maximum heart rate is 200. If you are 60, it is 160. This formula is derived from the observation that for each year you live your heart loses about a beat a minute.

The "target heart rate," as it is called in cardiovascular exercise programs, is pegged at about 70 to 85 percent of your maximum heart rate. Because everyone's heart and overall physiology is different, an individual's target heart rate is normally described as falling within a target heart rate range. The chart at the end of this chapter gives the maximum heart rate, the target heart rate, and the target heart rate range for ages 20 through 70 in five-year increments. You can calculate your own rate and range if your age falls between the ages listed.

Your Target Heart Rate Range

Maintaining your target heart rate is the key to the CONSUMER GUIDE® Aerobic Dancing Program. Your maximum heart rate is the greatest number of beats per minute that it can attain. During exercise, your heart rate should be approximately 75 percent of this maximum. To obtain the cardiovascular benefits of aerobic dancing—or of any other exercise—maintain a heart rate between 70 and 85 percent of your maximum heart rate for at least 15, or preferably 20, minutes. If you exceed 85 percent of your maximum, you are overdoing it and should relax your pace.

Just as important as it is to reach your target heart rate, it is vital not to exceed it. If you find you are reaching 90 percent or more of your maximum heart rate, you are overdoing. How will you know you are overdoing? Simple. Take your pulse while you are exercising.

By taking your pulse, you can check your heart rate while you dance. If you are at your target heart rate level—fine. If below, you must move more vigorously. If your pulse rate is above, do the exercises less vigorously.

Suppose you just finished a routine, and your pulse rate exceeded 90 percent of your maximum heart rate. Obviously you did the routine too vigorously. Next time don't raise your feet as high when you run in place, or perhaps you should walk in place instead. Learn to use your pulse rate as a guide to tell you whether you're getting enough exercise. It will take a little experimenting at first, but after a while you will be able to tell if you are within your range by the way you feel.

If you are tiring quickly or noticeably and you are exercising within your target heart rate range, you should reassess your range and lower it. Slow down until you are still working hard but not overextending yourself. If, on the other hand, you do not feel the effects of your dancing, you may not be exercising up to your true target rate.

You can determine if you are within your target heart rate range by placing three fingers over the artery near the center of the inside wrist. Touch three fingers lightly to that area until you can feel your pulse. Using a stopwatch or the second hand on a wristwatch or clock, count the number of beats for a period of 15 seconds. Then multiply this number by four to get your heart rate in beats per minute.

If you have difficulty in locating the pulse in your wrist—nothing to be alarmed about—you can find your heart rate by placing two or three fingers along your neck about one inch below the top of your jawbone and going through the same procedure.

An Aerobic Dance Workout

Our aerobic dancing program has three aims: to help you have fun, to condition your heart and lungs, and to improve your appearance. This dancing program will take you through progressive stages of conditioning. The conditioning goals are met naturally and automatically as you progress through the program. Your advance should be easy and comfortable, in step with your own body's demands.

As stated earlier, an aerobic exercise workout must have three periods—a warm-up, peak work, and a cool-down. The warm-up is a series of slow, methodical exercises which prepares the ligaments, tendons, and muscles for more vigorous movement. Warm-up exercises also prepare the heart, lungs, and blood vessels by increasing heart rate. The warm-up phase of the exercise program lasts about five to 10 minutes.

After the warm-up, peak work begins. Peak work is vigorous exercise which challenges your circulatory system and trains your heart and lungs to work more efficiently, bringing more oxygen to the body with less effort. To do this, you exercise vigorously enough to raise your pulse rate to somewhere between 115 and 170 beats per minute. You maintain that rate for a minimum of 15 minutes, and preferably for 20 minutes or longer.

At the conclusion of the peak work, you start a cool-down. The cool-down is really the warm-up in reverse. Like the warm-up, the cool-down is a series of slow, stretching exercises. About five to 10 minutes are devoted to the cool-down, which returns your body to more normal activity levels.

Let's look at each segment of a workout.

The Warm-Up

Professional dancers and athletes always warm-up before performing. They know that to perform well they must prepare their muscular, skeletal, and cardiovascular systems adequately.

Like other forms of vigorous exercise, aerobic dance requires a pre-exercise warm-up because it places stress on the human body. In order to withstand such stress, muscles must be made loose and flexible and blood circulation must be increased appreciably.

There are two effective methods of warming up: general calisthenics, which emphasizes stretching, and dance routines, which highlight stretching and slow movements. CONSUMER GUIDE® magazine recommends you do both, and our warm-up routines are designed to combine these two techniques.

Many aerobic dancers find the warm-up exercises to be less stimulating than peak work routines. Don't neglect the warm-up. It is an important and essential element in any workout.

The Cool-Down

The cool-down is the warm-up in reverse. After completing a strenuous exercise session you should help your body return to normal slowly. During the cool-down you want to keep your body in motion, but in low gear. Do some stretching exercises and slow dance routines. Or you can walk at a slow pace.

Neglecting the cool-down after a period of peak work can result in light-headedness, dizziness, nausea, or even fainting. You must let your body slowly return to its normal activity levels.

When you are exercising vigorously, your heart is rapidly pumping blood through the arteries so that it can supply active muscles with oxygen and life-supporting nutrients. The blood is forcefully pumped into the muscles by the contractions of the heart. There is, however, no similar force to send the blood back from the muscles to the heart by way of the veins.

If you abruptly stop exercising, blood begins to pool in the muscles and veins. A gradual tapering off, however, helps the muscles relax and aids the return of blood to the heart. The contracting leg muscles help "milk the blood" upward against gravity. More blood is returned to the heart and, consequently, to the brain, lessening the danger of light headedness and fainting.

The cool-down also helps your body in another way. Fatigue from exercise creates a build-up of a waste product, lactic acid, in the muscles. Cooling off may help dissipate the lactic acid and, therefore, ease muscle aches and pains.

A word of caution regarding the cool-down. Do not go into a sauna, a whirlpool bath, or hot shower until your heart rate has slowed to around 80 or 90 beats per minute. Even then—when cool-down is complete—avoid the steam room. It will not prevent aches and pains; it will not produce any permanent weight loss; and in some instances it can actually pose a health hazard. A shower is fine—but only after some tapering-off exercises. Even then, be sure to keep the water no hotter than lukewarm.

Warm-Up/Cool-Down Dance Routines

CONSUMER GUIDE® magazine recommends that you start your aerobic dance program by learning our warm-up/cool-down routines. You'll begin and end every workout with some of these routines, and learning them first will start conditioning your body for the more vigorous work ahead.

Spend at least one session in learning each routine. Take the following steps to learn each routine properly.
1. Listen to the record. That will give you a "feel" for a particular piece of music.
2. Read the directions for the specific routine.
3. Practice doing the routine without music.
4. "Walk through" the choreographed steps with the music.
5. Put the music and steps together.
Remember, don't aim for perfection when doing these routines; just keep your body moving and have a good time.

This procedure may take you 15 to 20 minutes, but it's the best way to learn a routine. Be patient. After you get the idea, you may be able to learn a three-minute routine in six to 10 minutes.

Peak Work

It's during the peak work that you get your whole body moving; your heart pumps faster; your rate of metabolism increases; you work at your target heart rate. Your muscles demand more oxygen, and your heart, lungs, and blood vessels supply them with sufficient quantities. Peak work is the most important part of your workout. It is during the peak work that calories are burned, fat is metabolized, the heart and lungs are conditioned, and tensions are released.

In this book, three levels of peak work are provided for you—low-intensity, moderate-intensity, and high-intensity. We have provided 10 peak-work routines. Don't try to learn all 10 routines at one time.

Learn the peak work routines as you did the warm-up/cool-down routines: (1) listen to the music; (2) read the directions; (3) try the various steps; (4) walk through the routine with the music; and (5) put the routine to music. Try to do the routines at a sufficient intensity to get your heart rate up to around 120 to 140 beats per minute.

You should spend a minimum of one day learning each of the four low-intensity peak work routines.

Putting It All Together

After you have learned the four low-intensity routines, you will be ready to do your first aerobic dance workout. An aerobic dance routine is a set of steps choreographed to one piece of music, i.e., "The Way We Were," "Le Freak," etc. An aerobic dance workout is a series of aerobic dance routines put together into a proper sequence of warm-up, peak work, and cool-down. A workout lasts about 30 minutes and should include a peak work segment of at least ten to 15 minutes.

Use two of the warm-up/cool-down routines for your warm-up session. Follow with the low-intensity routines, and complete your workout with the two remaining warm-up/cool-down routines. You should spend a minimum of two weeks with this low-intensity routine. During the next week you can begin to learn moderate-intensity routines, learning no more than one new routine during each workout.

Within a few weeks your peak work should consist of the moderate-intensity routines combined with two of the low-intensity routines. When you are ready for a new challenge, substitute learning one of the high-intensity routines for a low-intensity routine. As your routines become more vigorous, you can substitute a low-level routine for your warm-up/cool-down.

Vary your workouts by doing the routines in different orders. A low-intensity workout would be routines #1, #2, #7, #6, #5, #8, #4, and #3. A moderate routine could be: #3, #4, #7, #9, #11, #10, #5, #6, and #1. A high level workout could include: #1, #8, #9, #13, #12, #14, #11, #7, and #4.

Questions You May Have About the Program

How do I know I'm ready to progress to a more intense workout?

It depends upon your personal feelings and target heart rate. If you no longer find the workouts at a particular level challenging and if you find it increasingly difficult to get your heart rate up to its target level, it's time to move on.

When is the best time to learn a routine from the next level?

Right before the cool-down. Let's say that you've been working on the low-intensity aerobic dance workout. Before the cool-down take time to learn one new moderate-intensity routine. Spend at least a day learning the new routine.

What do I do between records?

Walk in place while you're waiting for the record

to change. If you want to do something more vigorous, you can run in place, hop in place, or practice a step you're unsure of. A pulse check is okay occasionally.

How well do I have to learn the routines?

Learn the routines as well as you want to. The purpose of aerobic dance is not perfection of skills but keeping your heart rate at its target level, burning calories, and enjoying yourself. Naturally, some of you will want to perfect dancing skills. That's okay. But remember, the real goal is movement and fun.

Why does my pulse rate seem to fluctuate so much?

Usually, your pulse rate jumps because you "really get into a routine," and let yourself go. Other times you are less sure of yourself, and you move more cautiously. You can solve this problem by trying to keep your body moving even if you "flub" or miss a step.

How many calories will I burn with this program?

For every 10 minutes you are at your target-heart-rate level you are burning 80 to 120 calories—about eight to 12 calories per minute—depending on your weight. If you weigh 125, you will burn about 80 calories; if you weigh 150, you'll burn about 100 calories; and if you weigh 175, you'll burn about 120 calories.

You can use this concept to "guesstimate" how much exercise you need to lose weight. First, estimate your caloric imbalance. If you are five pounds overweight, you are out of balance by 50 calories per day; 10 pounds, 100 calories; 15 pounds, 150 calories, etc. You simply add a zero to the number of pounds you'd like to lose, and this will give you the approximate number of calories you are out of balance. Remember, for every 100 calories you are out of balance you will need approximately 10 minutes of target-heart-rate exercise.

Will this kind of program really help me lose fat?

The longer you exercise, the more fat you will use. You don't have to worry about intensity as much as about duration. Fat is lost in the long run.

At rest, most of your energy comes from the carbohydrates which are stored in your body. In such intense activities as sprinting, swimming in races, and extremely vigorous dancing, practically all of your energy comes from glycogen. Those activities usually last less than a few minutes. But if you are able to engage in exercise lasting about 30 minutes, 50 percent of your energy will come from glycogen and the other 50 percent from fat. Sustained activities such as walking, jogging, swimming, and moderate dancing produce this result.

If the exercise lasts longer, fat stores on your body will supply almost 90 percent of the energy. So, if you have a problem with your body weight and fat, you want to make sure that your dance routines are longer rather than more intense.

What about spot reducing exercise?

Aerobic dance is an excellent way to remove unsightly bulges. It is far more effective than calisthentics or "stop-and-go" exercise.

If spot reducing worked, people who talked a lot would have thin faces. Research conducted at the University of California illustrates this point. The investigators studied the arms of tennis players who had been playing tennis at least six hours a week two years or more. Obviously, one arm of the tennis player had been subjected to more exercise than the other. If spot reducing worked, the exercised arm would have been thinner than the other one. But when doctors investigated the players they found the same amount of fat on each arm.

Does that mean I don't have to do spot reducing exercises?

It's not that the "spot reducing" exercises aren't good for you, it's just that they're inefficient in burning calories and removing fat. "Spot reducing" exercises are effective in firming and strengthening the muscles, but they're not likely to make you lose inches in specific areas. Spot reducing is physiological hogwash.

The beauty of aerobic dancing is that it is target-heart-rate exercise that helps you condition your heart and lungs as well as reduce body fat. In addition, you'll do many movements which strengthen and firm muscle groups. It's a true triple threat: exercise for the most important muscle in your body—your heart; exercise to reduce your body fat so you can see the muscles of your body; and exercise to strengthen different muscle groups to give your body nice form.

But won't stronger muscles make me look unsightly?

No. Behind every curve there is a muscle. An attractive shape is based on well-formed muscles. You won't have bulging biceps as a result of the aerobic dance program. It will give you a beautiful shape. Look at the dancers on television. Everyone would like to have their figures. Their muscles don't bulge. Muscles give the dancers their form and shape.

One last question. What happens when I have learned all the routines?

Move onto the last chapter. There we will tell you how to do your own thing.

Age	Your Maximum Heart Rate (beats per minute)	Your Target Heart Rate (75 percent of the maximum in beats per minute)	Your Target Heart Rate Range (between 70 percent and 85 percent of the maximum in beats per minute)
20	200	150	140 to 170
25	195	146	137 to 166
30	190	142	133 to 162
35	185	139	130 to 157
40	180	135	126 to 153
45	175	131	123 to 149
50	170	127	119 to 145
55	165	124	116 to 140
60	160	120	112 to 136
65	155	116	109 to 132
70	150	112	105 to 128

Sprains, Strains, Twitches, And Stitches

If you haven't exercised for some time, the stretching, hopping, and kicking of your aerobic dance program may cause your body to rebel. You may find yourself suffering sore muscles, strains, sprains, or any of a number of different aches and pains.

If you follow the go-slow program advocated in this book your chances of getting injured or hurt are greatly reduced. But problems can crop up in spite of the most cautious approach. However, most aches and pains are not serious and can be treated with a little rest and patience.

Achilles Tendinitis

One of the most common problems among aerobic dancers is a pain in the calf or the Achilles tendon. The Achilles tendon is the thick tendon at the back of the leg that connects the heel and foot to the back of the calf muscle. It controls the up-and-down motion of the foot and must stretch and contract a great deal to accommodate hopping and jumping movements.

Tendinitis, an inflammation of the tendon, should not be confused with the leg or calf pain that most people experience during the first few weeks of aerobic dance. Tendinitis has distinct symptoms: pain and stiffness an hour or so after activity;

swelling; pain on contraction and stretching of the calf muscles; and extreme tenderness to pressure applied to the tendon's narrowest point.

People who have worn high heels most of their life are especially susceptible to tendinitis. Wearing high heels for long periods compresses the calf muscles. Dance movements force them to stretch out, sometimes excessively, causing an inflammation of the tendon.

If you have tendinitis, put ice or cold water on the injured area. Cut back your activities to the point where the pain is tolerable. If the pain gets worse as you continue to exercise, you may have to stop until the condition improves.

As soon as you think that your Achilles tendon may be injured, avoid stretching it at all costs. Do not do the aerobic routines that focus on stretching. Pain is due to overstretching, and you must move slowly and avoid further strain.

To prevent tendinitis do the aerobic dance stretching routines in the warm-up and cool-down phases of your workout. You can also try adding a heel lift to your exercise shoes.

Shin Splints

Shin splints are pain felt in the front of the shin when you put weight on the ball of your foot. If you have a shin splint, your shin will be tender to the touch. In some cases, you may feel a roughened area along the bone when you run your fingers along the shin. Possible causes include:

1. An imbalance of muscles caused by a "toeing out" of the feet or other improper body mechanics.
2. A fracture (hairline) of one of the bones in the lower leg.
3. An inflammation of the tendon which is attached to the bone on the front of the lower leg.
4. A tearing of the tendon or muscle from the shinbone.
5. An irritation of the membrane between the two bones of the lower leg.
6. A dropping of the arch which irritates one or more of the tendons of the lower leg.
7. A weakening of the muscles in the front of the leg in comparison to the muscles at the back of the leg.

To prevent shin splints wear a good pair of shoes with a well-cushioned sole and a low heel when dancing. Running shoes are probably the best choice. Try to dance on as soft a surface as possible.

It's also a good idea to condition the muscles in the front of the leg. For example, try flexing your foot up and down against resistance. If you don't have weights handy to strap on your feet, sit with your feet dangling. Have a friend hold your feet while you try to pull your toes up. Do this 10 times, three times a day. If, despite your preventive efforts, you get shin splints, make sure that you put a sponge heel pad in your shoe to absorb some of the stress. You might even try a molded crest under your toes. If the pain is intolerable, try to avoid rising up on your toes.

Muscle Soreness and Stiffness

At one time or another we've all experienced sore or stiff muscles. This soreness or stiffness usually occurs 24 to 48 hours after engaging in vigorous exercise, and the pain generally lasts for only a few days. After severe exercise, it may last for a week. The most commonly affected muscles are those of the calves, back, thighs, and buttocks.

Experts do not agree on what causes sore and stiff muscles. Pain during and immediately following exercise is probably due to waste products formed during exercise and left in the fluids that surround the cells. Stiffness which occurs one to two days after exercise may be the result of small tears in muscle fibers or localized contractions of muscles.

It's almost impossible to avoid muscle soreness and stiffness completely, but you can reduce the intensity of pain by following our aerobic dancing program carefully, especially during the early

stages of exercise. A go-slow approach will allow the muscles of the body to adapt themselves to the stress placed upon them. If you do become sore and stiff, some additional light exercise or general activity will often provide temporary relief, but the pain usually returns when you stop. Longer cool-downs will help to avoid muscle soreness. Massage can also be beneficial. If the pain is severe, try applying ice packs.

Muscle Cramps and Spasms

After a heavy dancing session you may experience painful muscle contractions. Usually the pain occurs without warning, but occasionally you'll feel a cramp starting to build up. Cramps seem to occur most frequently at night.

The most common causes of muscle cramps are fatigue; cold; imbalance of salt, potassium, and water levels; a sharp blow; or an overstretching of unconditioned muscles. The cramps that you usually get at night after a heavy exercise session are brought about by a combination of fatigue and an overstretching of unconditioned muscles.

You can avoid muscle cramps by maintaining a good diet, making sure you warm-up properly prior to vigorous activity, and completing the routine with a cool-down. Try to work at a pace at which you will not become extremely fatigued.

When a cramp does occur it usually can be relieved by stretching and kneading the affected muscle. After the cramp goes away you may feel tightness or dull pain in the muscle area. When this happens, apply heat and massage to the area to restore circulation.

If you're plagued with frequent cramps, drink plenty of fluids and eat foods high in salt and potassium. You should also do muscle strengthening and stretching exercises.

Strains

Strains, also known as "pulled muscles" or "pulled tendons," are caused by overstretching a muscle or tendon. A sharp pain or "stitch" at the moment of injury is evidence of a pulled muscle or tendon. Dancers suddenly come up lame when they have pulled a muscle in their leg. The stiffness and soreness frequently worsens for two to three hours after the injury.

Moving the area affected by a strained muscle or tendon is quite painful, and the best treatment is to sit or lie in the most comfortable position, applying cold during the first 24 to 48 hours. After that, application of heat in any convenient form (heat lamp, hot water bottle, electric heating pad, etc.) and gentle massage to the painful area with warm rubbing alcohol is helpful.

When the soreness lessens, you can resume exercising. But you should do so gradually and cautiously. Most pulled muscles and tendons will heal with no more treatment than rest and a little patience on your part.

Sprains

Sprains are often confused with strains, but they are quite different. A strain is a pulled muscle or tendon. A sprain, on the other hand, is the stretching or tearing of ligaments which hold bones together at a joint. Any joint can be sprained: finger, wrist, shoulder, knee, ankle, or toe. The most common sprains—those of the ankle and knee—are the ones that will most often force you to curtail your aerobic dancing program.

Frequently, the average person cannot distinguish between a sprain and a fracture; even a doctor may not be able to tell without X-rays. Sometimes both sprain and fracture can result from the same injury. If you are unsure, check with your doctor.

Symptoms of a sprain include intense pain in the joint (the pain increases when the joint is touched or moved), rapid swelling, and often a black-and-blue discoloration which may not appear until several hours after the sprain.

Sprain prevention consists of precaution. If you're going to dance, be sure the floor is free of objects over which you could trip, thereby causing a sprain.

If you do sprain an ankle, try a technique doctors call ICE. The letters stand for Ice, Compression, and Elevation. Elevate your ankle higher than the rest of your body, apply ice, and give your ankle some support.

The compression or support you give your sprain may be a support bandage. To apply, place the middle of the elastic bandage under your foot, in front of the heel; cross ends in front, over the instep, and at the back of the heel; loop each end under the bandage and tie over the instep.

Once sprained, an ankle is very susceptible to spraining again. You may have to tape your ankle to give it additional support. You should also strengthen it through exercise. Some of the exercises in CONSUMER GUIDE® magazine's *The Complete Guide To Building A Better Body* will be helpful in strengthening an ankle.

Knee sprains can be serious and extremely painful. If you sprain your knee, get off the leg immediately and consult a doctor. The doctor will probably recommend ice packs and may immobilize the leg by splinting it or putting it in a cast.

Rest a sprained knee until the doctor allows you to renew your aerobic dancing program. And during exercise sessions you must be certain to avoid exercises which require full squatting. Consult *The Complete Guide To Building A Better Body* for exercises to strengthen an injured

knee after it has mended.

Above all, don't get impatient with strains and sprains. If you overwork the injured part, you run a high risk of reinjuring it and doing more harm than the original injury.

Dizziness

Dizziness is not an ache or pain, but it's a very important warning signal. If you become dizzy while exercising, stop immediately. Try to breathe normally and deeply. Dizziness may be due to overexertion.

Dizziness can also indicate the early stages of heat exhaustion or heat stroke, especially if you're exercising in a hot, humid room. When accompanied by shortness of breath, dizziness may be your body's warning of circulatory difficulties or other major medical problems. It may be a symptom of an equilibrium problem.

Try to wait out the dizzy spell. When you begin to feel better start exercising again, slowly and carefully. The dizziness may disappear as quickly as it came, but if it persists, stop exercising and see your doctor.

Pain in the Chest, Arms, etc.

While CONSUMER GUIDE® magazine's aerobic dance program is designed to strengthen your heart, it is possible that the workouts may be excessive for you. Check with your doctor before starting the program.

Heart problems are signaled by extreme or persistent pain down the arms, in the chest, neck, head, ears, or upper abdomen. Very heavy pressure on your chest as though someone were sitting on it, or extreme tightness inside the center of your chest are also symptoms of coronary distress. Other warnings include feelings like indigestion or stuffiness high in your stomach or low in your throat. If you have symptoms like these, you should stop exercising and see your doctor.

An Ounce of Prevention

Most of the aches and pains associated with aerobic dance are preventable. Injuries occur most often because of carelessness, fatigue, or overexertion. By following the cautious approach suggested here, and by being careful to warm-up and cool-down adequately, you will avoid much possible discomfort.

Remember too, that CONSUMER GUIDE® magazine's aerobic dance program is good protection against many injuries and ailments common in everyday life. The dancer's toned body, strengthened muscles, and improved cardiovascular health will prevent many of the maladies which afflict the more sedentary person.

The Routines

On the following pages are 14 aerobic dance routines. These routines are done to specific pieces of music. Most are three to four minutes in length, and they are classified into warm-up/cool-down, low-intensity, moderate-intensity, and high-intensity categories. Learn these routines in sequence as they appear.

Start with the warm-up/cool-down routines. During the weeks to come, progress from the low-intensity routines into the moderate-, and high-intensity routines. This will allow your muscles, tendons, and ligaments to adjust to the vigorousness of the exercise and will prepare your circulatory system for more demanding levels of activity.

Remember, the idea behind aerobic dancing is to keep moving. That way, you'll burn more calories and keep your heart rate at its target level. It is more important to keep your body moving than it is to learn each step precisely. Don't hold up your fitness progress by trying to perfect a routine.

Seek your own level of activity when doing these routines. We haven't suggested a specific number of repetitions for each exercise in a routine. If we had, you might strain to reach that number and thereby exceed your target heart rate. Push yourself hard enough to challenge your circulatory system, but don't overextend yourself.

How To Read a Routine

We have divided the description of each routine into four segments: Music Cue, Beats, Action, and Picture Cue. Each heading has a specific meaning. The *Music Cue* is just that, a cue. It will tell you when you are to start a new exercise. *Beats* tells you how long you will be doing that particular exercise, whether for eight beats, or 16, or 32. *Action* tells you what exercise you will be doing, Kicks, or Side Hops, or Arm Swings for example. *Picture Cue* refers you to the sequence of pictures and text that tell you how to do the exercise.

Take, for example, routine number seven, "Two Doors Down" by Dolly Parton. The first line of instructions for this routine indicates that there are 32 beats (Beats) during the instrumental phase (Music Cue). During this time you will be doing Double Hip Bumps (Action). The photos in section

A (Picture Cue) will show you how to do the exercise.

Look to section A for complete directions for doing Double Hip Bumps. The text describes your starting position (SP), and then tells you to rock your hip to the right (R) twice, and then to the left (L) twice. (If a movement continues over several beats or should be held for a certain number of beats the text will specify that as well.)

Do the Double Hip Bumps at a rate with which you feel comfortable. Generally, 16 Double Hip Bumps could be done in this 32-beat segment of the record, but the number that you do depends on your ability and fitness level.

Let's move to the second line of instructions. When the Music Cue *Two doors down . . .* comes in, move into the Arrow Step (Action), which is described in Picture Cue B. Do this exercise for 32 beats. At the conclusion of this 32-beat segment, you'll hear the Music Cue *I think I'll . . .,* and you should do the Polka Step (third line), described in Picture Cue C. Again, this exercise is done for 32 beats. The number of Polka Steps that you'll do is contingent upon your ability. The Music Cue *Two doors down . . .* indicates that you then repeat the Arrow Step. Continue the sequence in this manner, always working at your own pace.

Just remember: The key is to move to the music and to move fast enough to reach your target heart rate. If you haven't been leading a very active life, you'll probably move less vigorously than someone who is very fit. The CONSUMER GUIDE® system allows you to tailor each aerobic dance routine to your fitness level, age, and general well-being.

Two Important Hints

1. You'll notice that our model occasionally stands at an angle to the camera. This was done so that you could better see details like arm and foot placement. But, unless our description of the exercise indicates otherwise, you should continue facing forward.

2. Once you have learned the routines, you will no longer need pictures. We suggest that you then write down the Music Cue, Beats, and Action on a card and file it. You can use these for handy reference to your aerobic dance routines.

1. The Way We Were

by Barbra Streisand   Columbia 13-33262

Let Barbra Streisand help stretch the muscles and tendons of your legs. Do all the moves slowly and deliberately. When stretching go to the point of discomfort—no further. Concentrate on relaxing. This routine promotes flexibility.

MUSIC CUE	BEATS	ACTION	PICTURE CUE
instrumental	4	Wait	
oooh . . .	8	Walk Down Legs	A
oooh . . hmm . . .	8	Hold Four; Walk Up Legs	B
humming	8	repeat Walk Down Legs	A
humming	8	repeat Hold Four; Walk Up Legs	B
Mem'ries light the . . .	8	Crossed Leg Walk Down	C
. . . of my mind . . .	8	Elephant	D
. . . color mem'ries of . . .	8	Elephant Reach	E
. . . we were.	8	Body Lean	F
Scattered pictures of . . .	8	repeat Crossed Leg Walk Down (opposite leg forward)	C
. . . left behind. Smiles . . .	8	repeat Elephant	D

MUSIC CUE	BEATS	ACTION	PICTURE CUE
. . . another for the . . .	8	repeat Elephant Reach	E
. . . way we were . . .	8	repeat Body Lean	F
Can it be . . .	32	Shoulder Stretch	G
Mem'ries may be . . .	8	repeat Crossed Leg Walk Down	C
. . . yet what's too . . .	8	repeat Elephant	D
. . . remember we simply . . .	8	repeat Elephant Reach	E
. . . forget. So it's . . .	8	repeat Body Lean	F
. . . laughter we will . . .	8	Arms Front	H
. . . remember whenever we . . .	8	Arms Side	I
. . . remember the way . . .	8	Arm Extensions	J
. . . were the way . . .	8	Arms Front & Side	K
. . . were . . . oooh . . .	8	repeat Walk Down Legs	A
. . . oooh . . .	4	repeat Hold Four	B
. . . oooh . . .	4	repeat Walk Up Legs	B
humming	5	repeat Walk Down Legs	A

A. Walk Down Legs

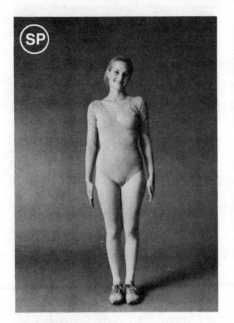

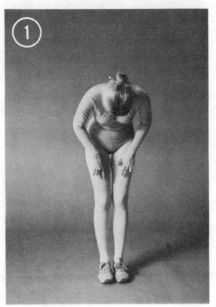

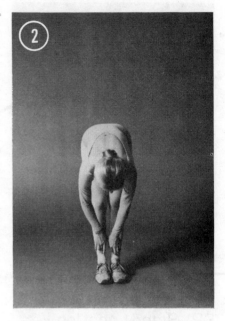

SP: Stand,
feet together.

1. Bend forward
at waist.

2. Walk fingers down
legs as far as possible.
(Takes 8 beats.)

B. Hold Four; Walk Up Legs

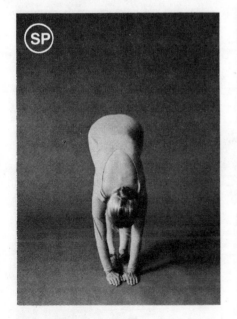

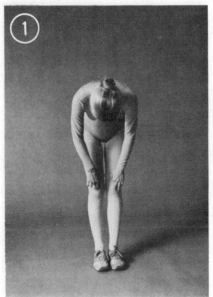

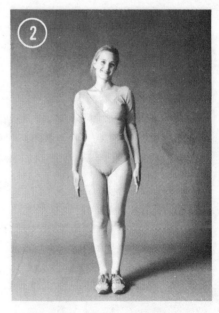

SP: Hold final
position from Walk
Down Legs for 4 beats.

1. Walk fingers up
legs. (Takes 4 beats.)

2. Bring upper body
to full upright
position.

C. Crossed Leg Walk Down

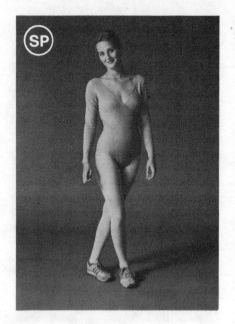

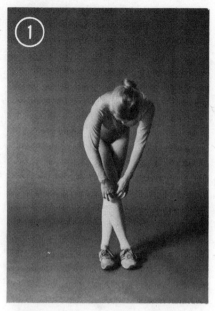

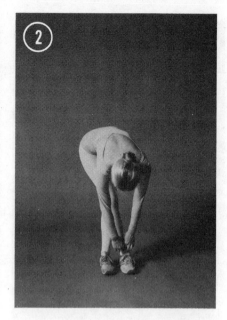

SP: Stand, one leg crossed over the other.

1. Bend forward from waist.

2. Walk fingers down leg. (Takes 8 beats).

D. Elephant

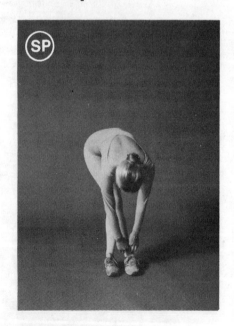

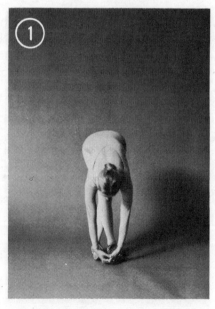

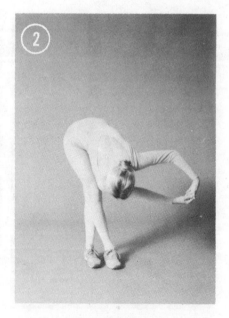

SP: Hold final position of Crossed Leg Walk Down.

1. Clasp hands.

2. Move R arm across body to the side keeping it straight. (Takes 3 Beats)

D. Elephant (Continued)

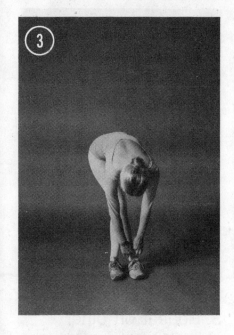

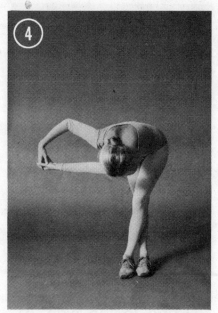

3. Return to SP.
(Takes 1 Beat)

4. Repeat on
other side.

E. Elephant Reach

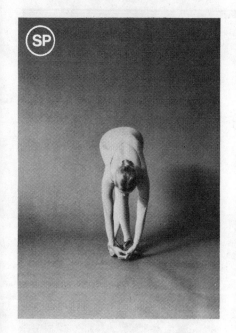

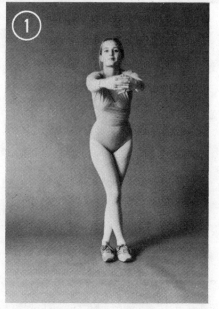

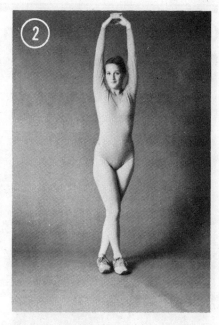

SP: Legs crossed,
upper body bent over,
hands clasped in front
of feet or shins.

1. Raise upper body,
stretching clasped
hands out in front of
body.

2. Continue until
clasped hands
are completely
extended above head.
(Takes 8 beats.)

F. Body Lean

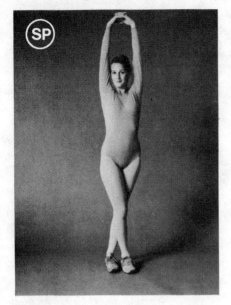

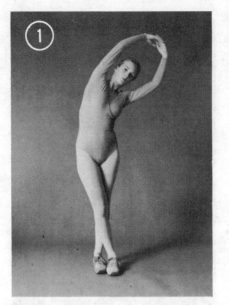

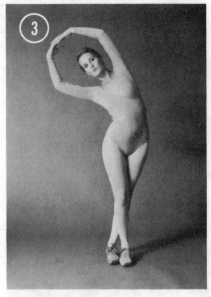

SP: Stand, arms
overhead and
feet crossed.

1. Bend to the side.
(Takes 3 Beats)
2. Return to SP.
(Takes 1 Beat)

3. Repeat on other
side. Keep hands
clasped throughout
movement.

G. Shoulder Stretch

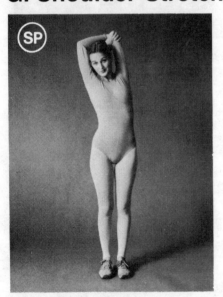

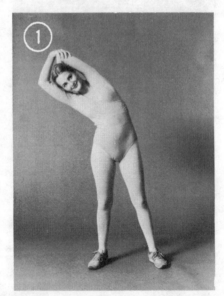

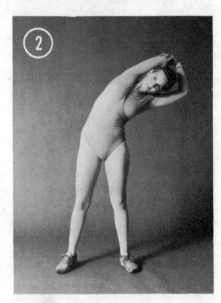

SP: Stand, L arm
bent behind head,
L hand on R shoulder.
Place R hand
on L elbow.

1. Gently pull L arm
over and down,
stretching L side.
(Takes 4 Beats) Return
to SP. (Takes 4 Beats)

2. Bend to R side.
Return and repeat
on opposite side.

H. Arms Front

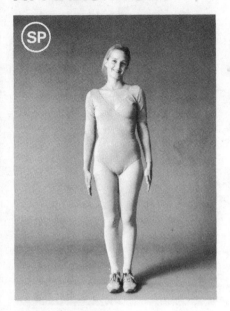 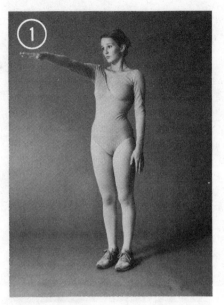 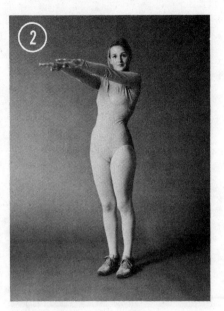

SP: Stand,
arms at sides.

1. Extend R arm
forward to chest
height; hold for 4 beats.

2. Extend L arm;
hold for 4 beats.

I. Arms Side

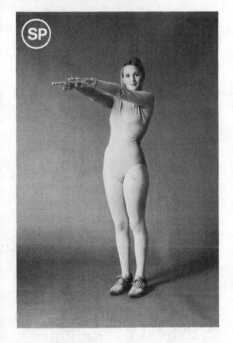 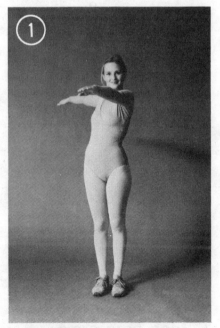 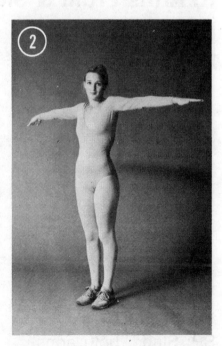

SP: Stand, both arms
extended in front.

1. Extend R arm to
side; hold for 4 beats.

2. Extend L arm to
side; hold for 4 beats.

J. Arm Extensions

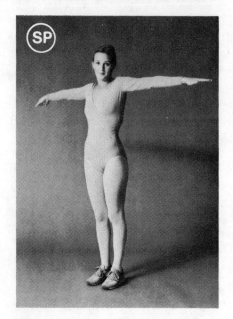 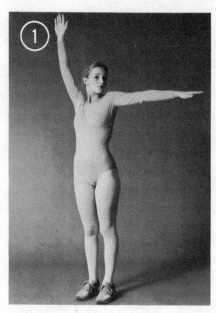 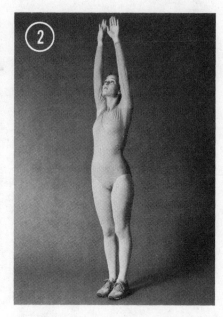

SP: Stand, arms extended to the sides at shoulder height.

1. Extend R arm upward above head; hold for 4 beats.

2. Extend L arm upward above head; hold for 4 beats.

K. Arms Front & Side

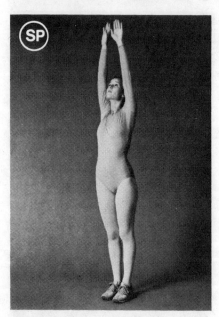 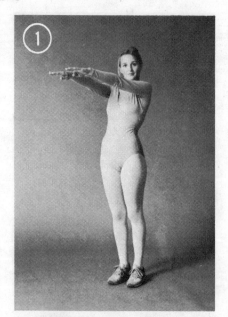 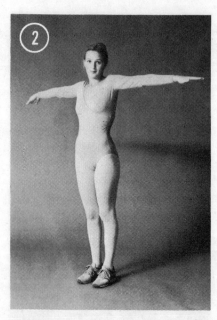

SP: Stand, both arms extended over head.

1. Bring both arms to front; hold for 4 beats.

2. Extend both arms to sides; hold for 4 beats.

2. Rock Around The Clock

by Bill Haley and The Comets   MCA-60025

What better way is there to warm up to exercise than with the originators of rock and roll—Bill Haley and The Comets. "Rock Around The Clock" will *wake up* your flaccid muscles, tendons, and ligaments. It will get you *in the groove* to move 24 hours a day.

MUSIC CUE	BEATS	ACTION	PICTURE CUE
One, two, three . . .	16	Clock Hands	
. . . glad rags on . . .	24	Heel-Toe Swing	
. . . clock strikes two . . .	24	Pendulum	
instrumental	24	Dig Step	
. . . chimes ring five . . .	24	repeat Heel-Toe Swing	
. . . eight, nine, ten . . .	24	repeat Pendulum	
instrumental	24	repeat Dig Step	
. . . clock strikes twelve . . .	24	repeat Heel-Toe Swing	
instrumental	4	repeat Clock Hands	

A. Clock Hands

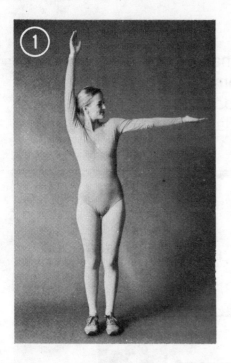 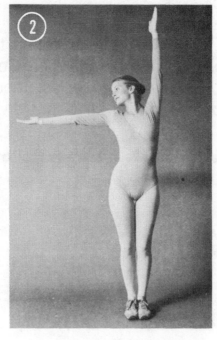

SP: Stand.

1. Extend R arm above head so that it is perpendicular to the floor. Simultaneously extend L arm to side, parallel to floor. Face L.

2. While keeping both arms straight, shift them so that the L arm is extended above head and R arm is extended to the side.

3. Continue shifting R and L.

B. Heel-Toe Swing

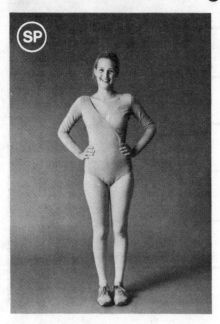 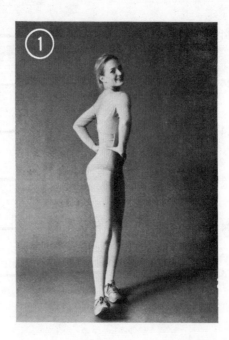

SP: Stand, hands on hips.

1. Walk, beginning with R foot. As R leg is extended, twist upper torso so R elbow points forward. Tap floor with R heel; point R toes up.

B. Heel-Toe Swing (Continued)

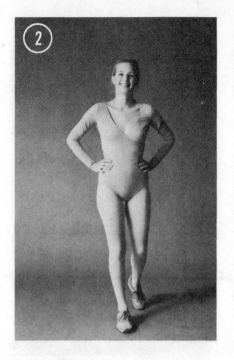

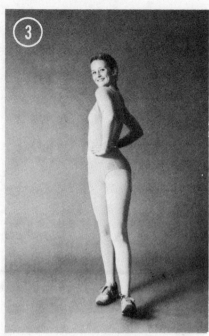

2. When R foot is completely flat on the floor and L heel is off the ground, turn upper torso to face front.

3. Repeat Step #1, beginning with L leg.

C. Pendulum

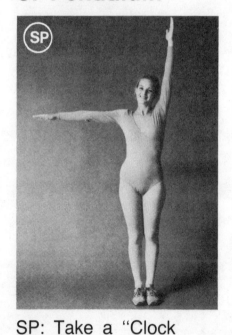

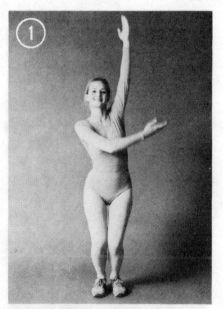

2. After second pendulum swing continue R arm up to 12 o'clock position. At same time L arm goes down into a pendulum swing. Swing L arm twice.

3. Continue, alternating direction of swing.

SP: Take a "Clock Hands" position

L arm at 12 o'clock perpendicular to the floor and R arm at 9 o'clock parallel to the floor.

1. Swing R arm like a pendulum down and across body twice. Bend the knees on each downward swing.

D. Dig Step

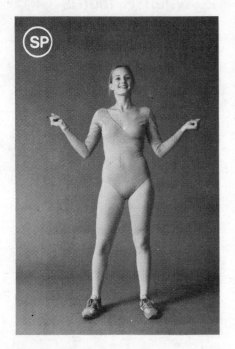

SP: Stand, arms at sides, elbows bent.

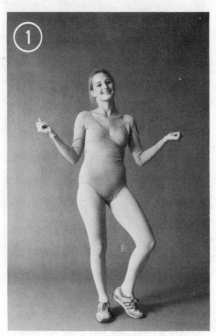

1. Tap the toes of L foot on floor close to R foot.

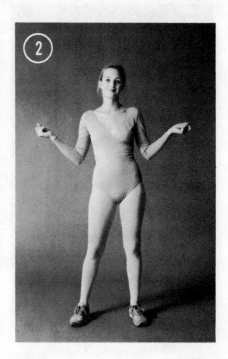

2. Step L foot to the L side.

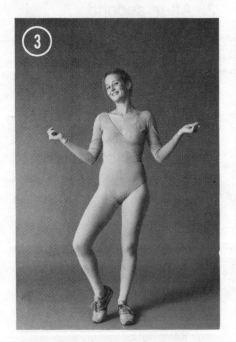

3. Bring R foot close to L foot, and tap the toes of R foot to floor.

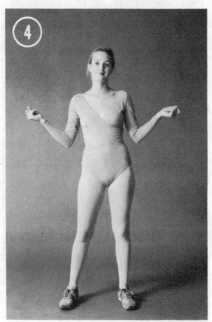

4. Step R foot to the R side.

not on tape

3. Talkin' In Your Sleep

warm-up/cool-down
time: 2:53

by Crystal Gayle   United Artists UA-X1214-Y

This warm-up/cool-down routine is done on the floor. It will prepare your muscles, tendons, and ligaments for practically any workout of any intensity. Try to do the exercises smoothly and without pause.

MUSIC CUE	BEATS	ACTION	PICTURE CUE
Three o'clock in . . .	11	Head Rolls	A
. . . listenin' to your . . .	16	Look Up	B
. . . haven't heard you . . .	16	Floor Jumping Jacks	C
. . . close your eyes . . .	16	Knee Raises	D
. . . sleep. Sleepin' in . . .	16	Cross Body Arm Swings	E
. . . tight lovin'; her . . .	16	Arm Bicycle Pumps	F
. . . sleep with lovin' . . .	16	Knee Lifts	G
. . . haven't heard you . . .	16	repeat Floor Jumping Jacks	C
. . . close your eyes . . .	16	repeat Knee Raises	D
. . . sleep. Sleepin' in . . .	16	repeat Cross Body Arm Swings	E
. . . tight lovin'; her . . .	16	repeat Arm Bicycle Pumps	F
. . . sleep with lovin' . . .	13	repeat Knee Lifts	

A. Head Rolls

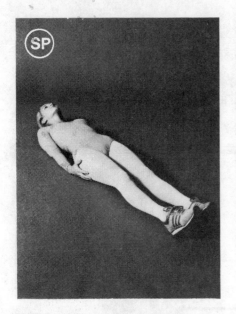 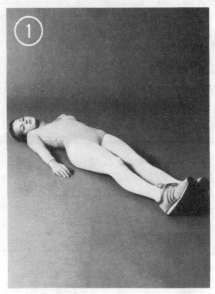 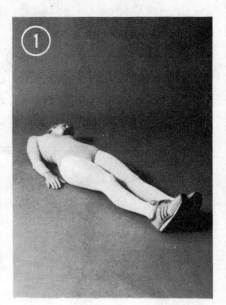

SP: Lie on floor, on your back, arms alongside body.

1. Roll head from R to L so each ear touches respective shoulder.

B. Look Up

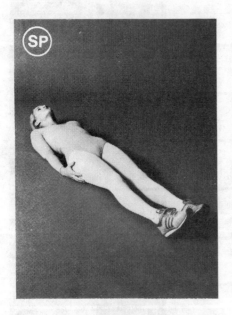 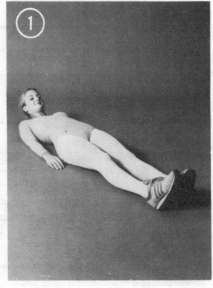

SP: Lie on floor, on your back, arms alongside body.

1. Curl head up off floor so chin comes toward chest. Return.

C. Floor Jumping Jacks

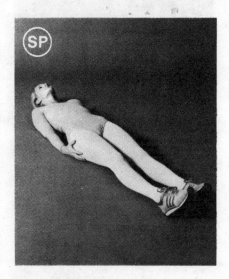

SP: Lie on floor, on your back, arms alongside body.

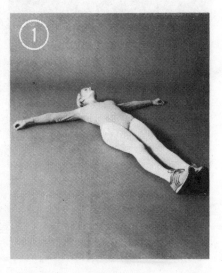

1. Slide arms along floor so they are perpendicular to the body. (beat 1)

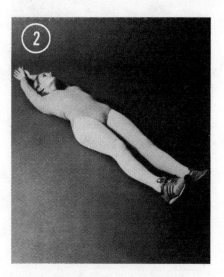

2. Continue to move arms above head until hands touch. (beat 2)

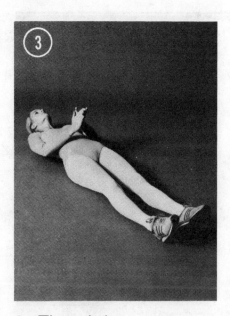

3. Then bring arms down in front of body and clap hands. (beat 3)

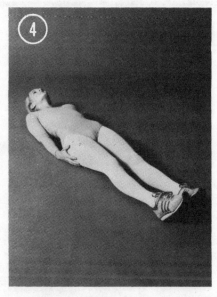

4. Return to SP. (beat 4)

D. Knee Raises

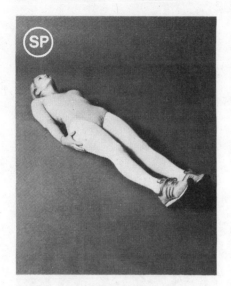 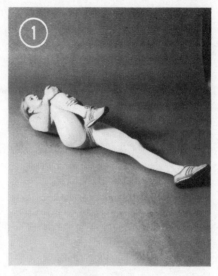 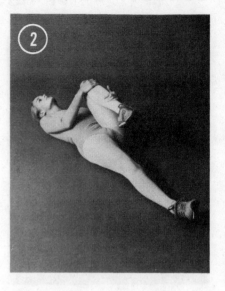

SP: Lie on floor, on your back, arms alongside body.

1. Raise R knee to chest. As knee comes to chest, grasp knee and shin with both hands. Return to SP.

2. Repeat on other side.

E. Cross Body Arm Swings

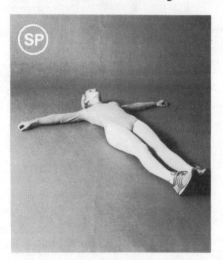 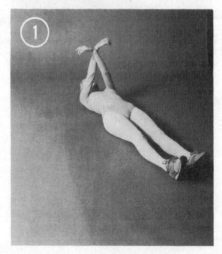 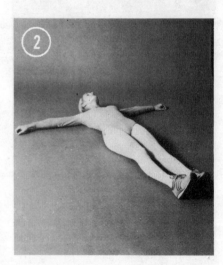

SP: Lie on back, arms extended at shoulders, perpendicular to body.

1. Keeping arms straight, bring them across the chest. Arms should cross at wrists, hands should be relaxed.

2. Return to SP.

34

F. Arm Bicycle Pumps

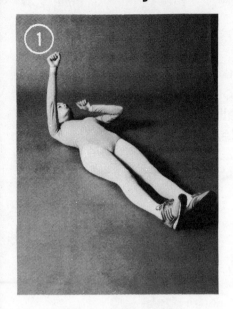 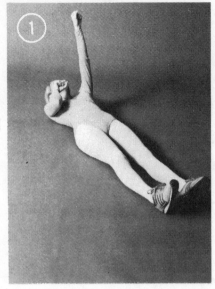

SP: Lie on back with arms raised in front of chest and bent at elbows.

1. Alternately extend the R and then the L arm. When one arm is extended, the other arm is bent. Continue pumping action.

G. Knee Lifts

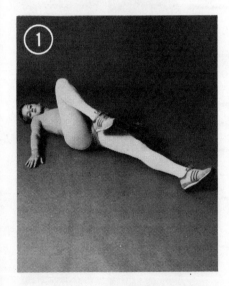 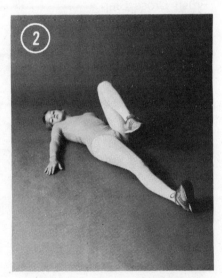 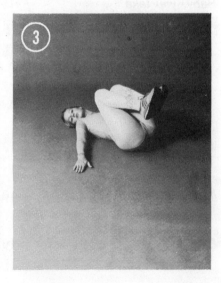

SP: Lie on back, arms extended to the side at a 45° angle from body.

1. Raise R knee up off floor and toward chest. Return. (Takes 2 Beats)

2. Raise L knee up toward chest, and return. (Takes 2 Beats)

3. Raise R knee; then L knee. Return R leg to floor; then L leg. (Takes 4 Beats)

4. I Just Fall In Love Again

by Anne Murray   Capital 4675

Warm-up/cool-down routines are designed to prepare your muscles, tendons, and ligaments for more vigorous exercise or to relax them after strenuous work. Do not do these rapidly. Do all warm-up/cool-down movements slowly. Stretch and allow the music to lead you.

MUSIC CUE	BEATS	ACTION	PICTURE CUE
instrumental	2	wait	
instrumental	14	Side Step Drag (3 times L, 4 times R)	
Dreamin', I must . . .	16	Halo	
Baby, you take . . .	16	Brush Cross Step	
. . . though, I just . . .	16	Thigh Brush Reach	
. . . go, I just . . .	16	Lunge Knee Raise	
instrumental	12	repeat Side Step Drag (4 times L, 2 times R)	
Magic, it must . . .	16	repeat Halo	
Easy for you . . .	16	repeat Brush Cross Step	
. . . though, I just . . .	16	repeat Thigh Brush Reach	
. . . go, I just . . .	16	repeat Lunge Knee Raise	
Can't help myself . . .	24	repeat Side Step Drag (4 times L, 4 times R, 4 times L)	

A. Side Step Drag

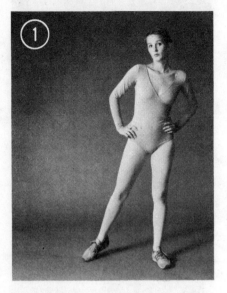 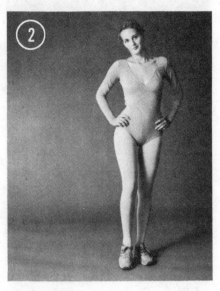 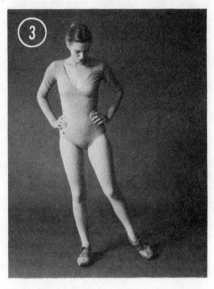

SP: Stand, hands on hips.
1. Step the L foot about 24" to the L. Shift weight to L foot.

2. Drag the R foot to meet the L foot.

3. Repeat as indicated in summary.

B. Halo

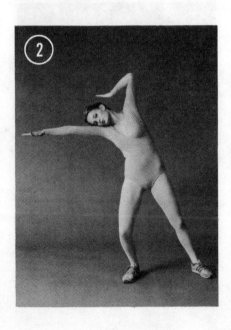 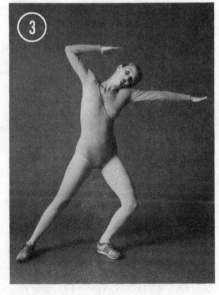

SP: Stand.

1. Extend R arm to side, parallel to the floor. Rest R side of head on R shoulder. The L arm should be bent at the elbow, palm facing the floor, L hand over the head. Make a circle over the head with the L hand,

2. Simultaneously shift the weight to the R leg and extend the L leg.

3. Repeat on opposite side.

C. Brush Cross Step

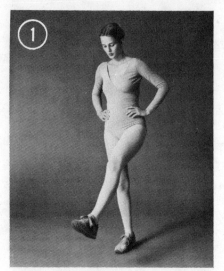 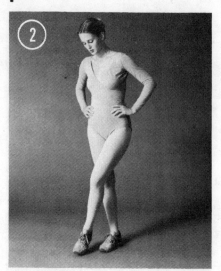 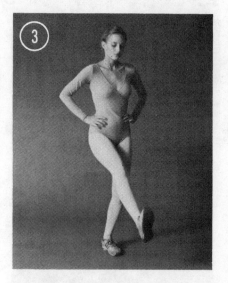

SP: Stand, hands on hips.

1. Shift all weight to the R foot, and brush L foot along the floor, kicking once.

2. Cross L foot in front of the R foot, and step L foot down to the side of the R foot, shifting weight to L foot.

3. Repeat on other side.

D. Thigh Brush Reach

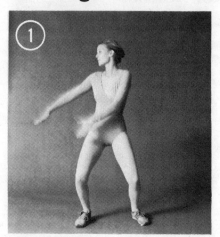 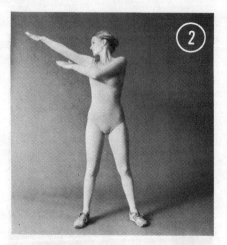 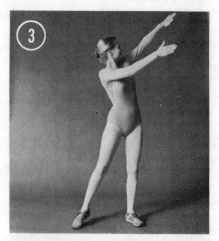

SP: Stand.

1. Bend the knees, and simultaneously brush both thighs with the hands, swinging arms to the R.

2. Continue swing until arms are at least parallel to the floor. At same time swing body upward so that arms are fully extended, knees straight.

3. Repeat on the other side.

E. Lunge Knee Raise

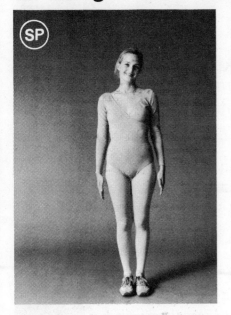
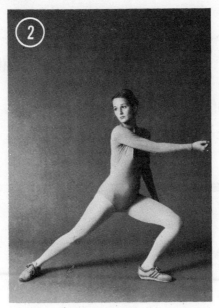

SP: Stand.

1. Shift weight to the L by bending the L knee and extending the R leg as shown.

2. As you shift to the L, swing the R arm down in an arc in front of the body and to the L.

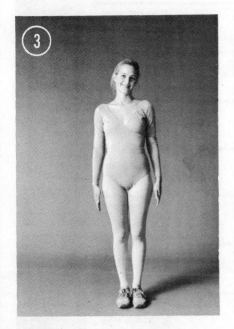
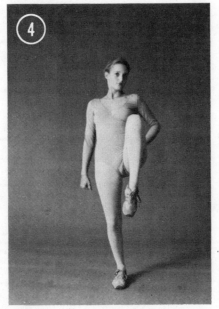
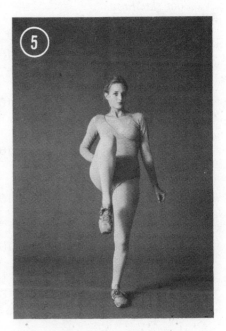

3. Return to the SP.

4. Now raise the L knee.

5. Return to the SP and repeat on other side.

5. Le Freak

by Chic   Atlantic 3519

low-intensity
time 3:30

You can get fit while you sit. Don't feel like a freak when you're doing this number. It's fun from the word "go." *Feel the rhythm* of the song as you move. Put yourself into it. The only reason this routine is considered low-intensity is that you sit through it.

MUSIC CUE	BEATS	ACTION	PICTURE CUE
One, two ah . . .	4	Sitting Claps	A
. . . out, Le Freak . . .	16	Sitting Alternate Heel-Toe Touches	B
. . . out, Le Freak . . .	16	Sitting Arm Flings	C
Have you heard . . .	16	Sitting Cheerleader	D
Big fun to . . .	16	Sitting Alternate Arm Raises	E
Young and old . . .	16	Sitting Side Hops	F
It's called Le . . .	16	Sitting Circle Snaps	G
. . . out. Le Freak . . .	16	Sitting Arm Switches	H
All that pressure . . .	16	Sitting Alternate Floor Touches	I
Feel the rhythm . . .	16	Sitting Alternate Leg Kicks	J
Like the days . . .	16	Sitting Knee Raises	K

MUSIC CUE	BEATS	ACTION	PICTURE CUE
Just come on . . .	16	Sitting Arm Swings	
. . . out, Le Freak . . .	16	repeat Sitting Arm Switches	
. . . freak. instrumental	32	Sitting Butterfly Taps	
instrumental	16	repeat Sitting Arm Flings	
instrumental	16	repeat Sitting Alternate Heel-Toe Touches	
. . . freak. instrumental	16	repeat Sitting Cheerleader	
instrumental	16	repeat Sitting Alternate Arm Raises	
. . . freak. instrumental	16	repeat Sitting Side Hops	
instrumental	16	repeat Sitting Circle Snaps	
All that pressure . . .	16	repeat Sitting Alternate Floor Touches	
Feel the rhythm . . .	16	repeat Sitting Alternate Leg Kicks	
Like the days . . .	16	repeat Sitting Knee Raises	
Just come on . . .	16	repeat Sitting Arm Swings	
. . . out, Le Freak . . .	32	repeat Sitting Arm Switches	

A. Sitting Claps

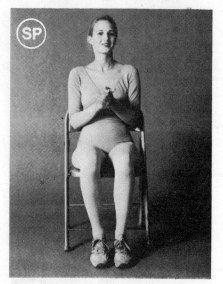

SP: Sit in a chair.

Clap hands in rhythm to the music.

B. Sitting Alternate Heel-Toe Touches

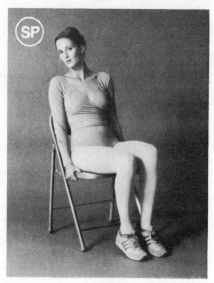

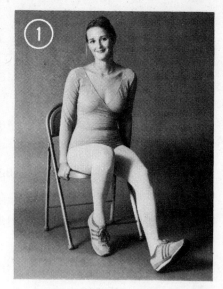

SP: Sit. Hold onto the sides of chair.

1. Alternately extend L and then R foot forward. When the leg is forward, the heel taps the floor. When leg is back, the toe taps the floor.

C. Sitting Arm Flings

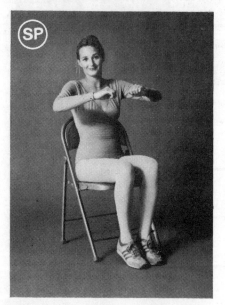

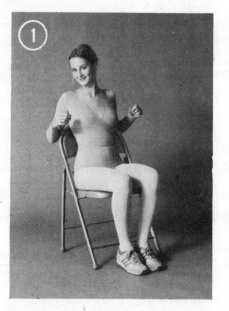

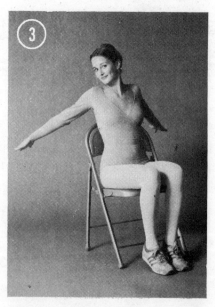

SP: Sit, arms bent at elbows, hands held in loose fists at chest height.

1. Push both elbows backward. (Takes 1 Beat)
2. Return to SP. (Takes 1 Beat)

3. Straighten arms and fling arms backward. (Takes 1 Beat)
4. Return to SP. (Takes 1 Beat)

D. Sitting Cheerleader

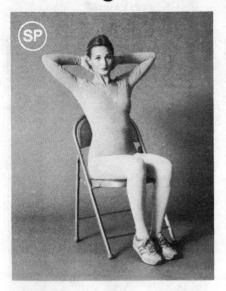

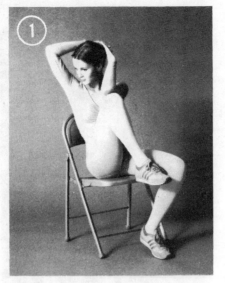

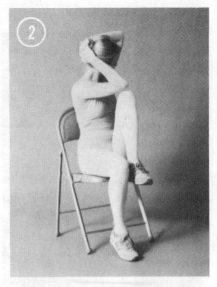

SP: Sit, hands clasped behind head.

1. Raise one knee, twist upper torso toward raised knee, touch opposite elbow to knee.

2. Return to SP. Repeat on other side.

E. Sitting Alternate Arm Raises

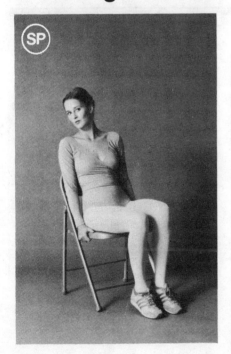

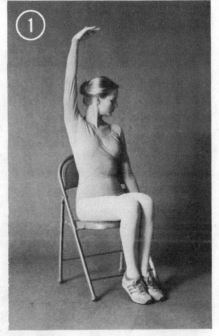

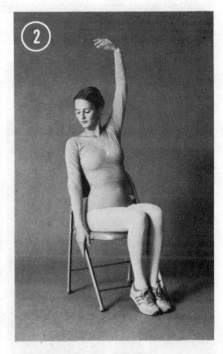

SP: Sit, arms at sides.

1. Raise R arm over head. (Takes 2 Beats)

2. Raise L arm over head, and lower R arm to side. (Takes 2 Beats)

F. Sitting Side Hops

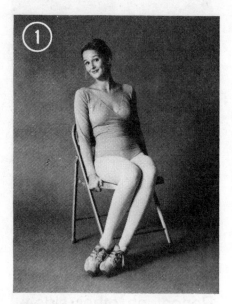

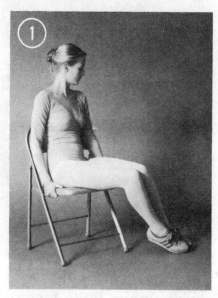

SP: Sit, holding onto sides of the chair.

1. Tap both toes to the R and then to the L.

G. Sitting Circle Snaps

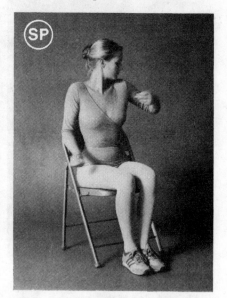

SP: Sit. With each beat describe a small circle with each hand. Snap fingers as you rotate hands.

H. Sitting Arm Switches

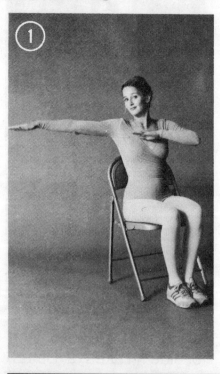

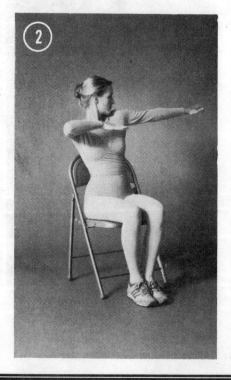

SP: Sit.

1. Extend R arm out to side while bringing L arm across chest. (Takes 2 Beats)

2. Extend L arm out to side while bringing R arm across chest. (Takes 1 Beat)

3. Return arms to R side. (Takes 1 Beat)

4. Repeat pattern, beginning on L side, holding for 2 beats.

I. Sitting Alternate Floor Touches

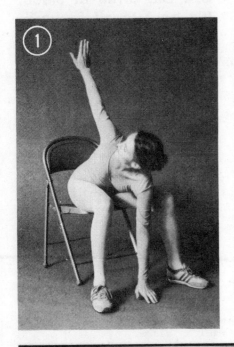
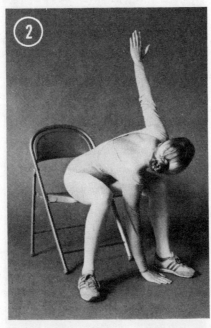

SP: Sit, feet on floor about 24" apart.

1. Bend forward and twist to R, extending R arm upward and backward. At same time touch L hand to floor between feet.

2. Twist to L and extend L arm upward and touch R hand to floor.

J. Sitting Alternate Leg Kicks

K. Sitting Knee Raises

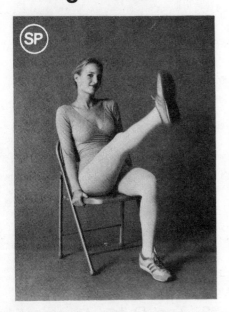
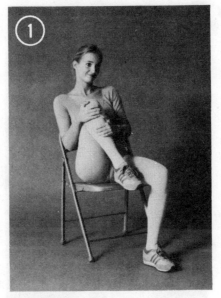
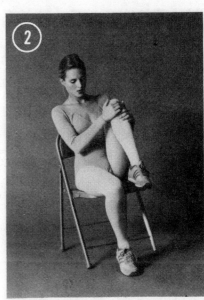

SP: Sit, holding onto sides of chair. Extend and kick R leg, return leg to floor, then L leg. Continue alternating.

SP: Sit.

1. Raise knee to chest, grasp knee and shin with both hands.

2. Return to SP and repeat on other side.

L. Sitting Arm Swings

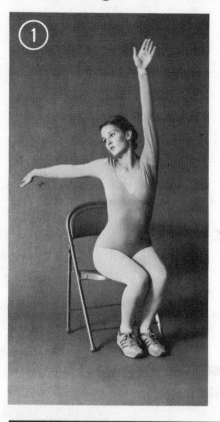 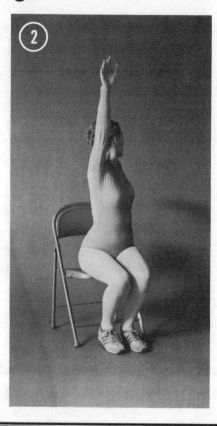

SP: Sit, arms at sides. It's best to sit forward on chair.

1. Swing R arm back and up, simultaneously swinging L arm to front and up.

2. Repeat on other side.

M. Sitting Butterfly Taps

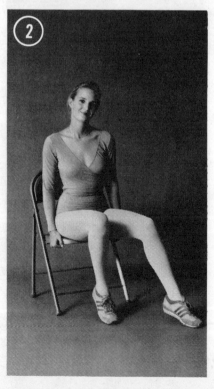 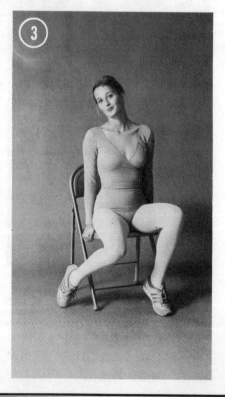

SP: Sit on edge of chair, holding onto sides, toes together in front of chair.

1. Tap R toe to front and bring back to SP.

2. Tap L toe to front and bring back to SP.

3. Tap R toe to side, and bring back to SP.

4. Tap L toe to side, and bring back to SP.

6. Thank You For Being A Friend

low-intensity
time 4:41

by Andrew Gold   Asylum 45087

Your body will thank you for doing this low-intensity aerobic dance routine. Move to the music, and don't stop between the various exercises. This is a bouncy number; let yourself respond to the rhythm. Because this routine has only five basic exercises you will be able to learn it quickly.

MUSIC CUE	BEATS	ACTION	PICTURE CUE
instrumental	8	Single Hip Bumps	A
Thank you for . . .	32	Around the World	B
I'm not ashamed . . .	32	Walk Reverse	C
And if you . . .	32	Hand Swing	D
. . . friend . . . thank you	32	Grapevine	E
instrumental . . .	8	repeat Around the World	B
If it's a . . .	32	repeat Walk Reverse	C
I'm not ashamed . . .	32	repeat Hand Swing	D
And when we . . .	32	repeat Grapevine	E
. . . friend . . . thank you	32	repeat Around the World	B
. . . friend . . . thank you	32	repeat Walk Reverse	C
. . . die and float . . .	32	repeat Hand Swing	D
. . . call as we . . .	32	repeat Grapevine	E

MUSIC CUE	BEATS	ACTION	PICTURE CUE
instrumental	32	repeat Around the World	
. . . *friend. I want* . . .	32	repeat Walk Reverse	
. . . *I want to* . . .	32	repeat Hand Swing	
. . . *tell you right* . . .	32	repeat Grapevine	
instrumental	9	repeat Single Hip Bumps	

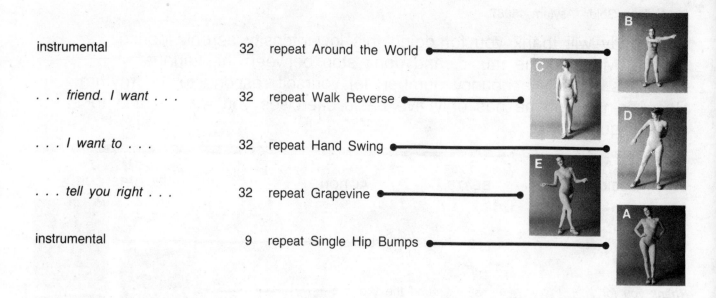

A. Single Hip Bumps

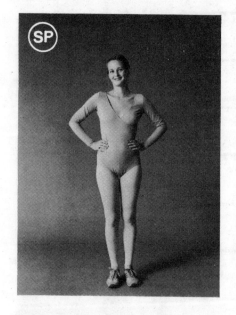

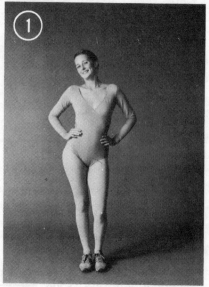

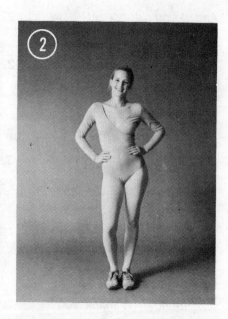

SP: Stand, hands on hips.

1. Rock R hip once to R.

When rocking, R knee is straight and L leg is bent slightly at the knee.

2. Rock L hip once to L.

B. Around the World

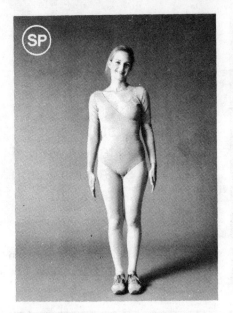

SP: Stand.

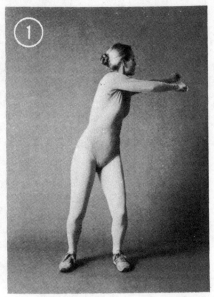

1. Reach out to the L side and back with both hands and snap fingers.

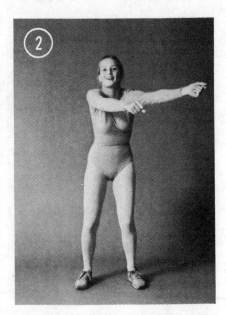

2. Bring arms across front of body, stretching arms as much as possible. Bend forward slightly, and continue snapping fingers.

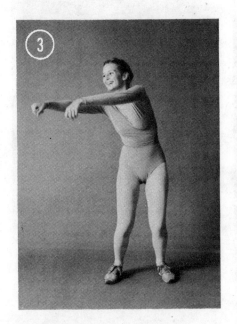

3. Continue bringing arms across chest toward the R, fingers snapping.

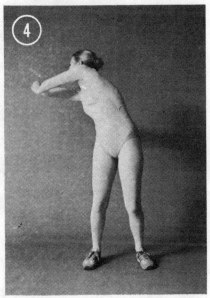

4. Reach back to the R as far as possible, and continue snapping.

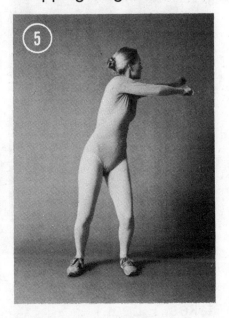

5. Quickly return to L. Repeat.

Note: Bend knees (bounce) slightly as arm pattern is performed.

C. Walk Reverse

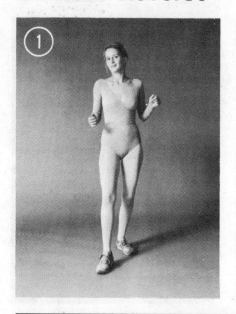

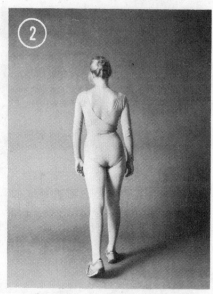

SP: Stand.

1. Walk 4 steps forward.

2. On 4th step turn about face, walk 4 steps in same direction as first 4 steps but facing backward.

Note: All 8 steps progress in the same direction, but you face backward the last 4 steps.

D. Hand Swing

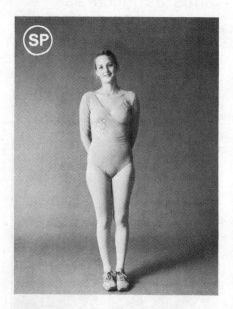

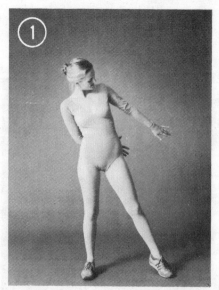

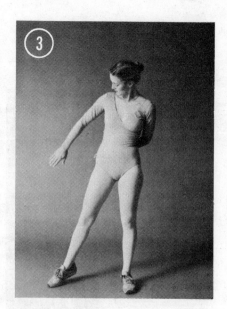

SP: Stand with arms behind back. (Each step in this exercise takes 1 beat.)

1. Touch L toe to the L side. Simultaneously swing arms to the L, R arm behind the back and L to the side.

2. Return to SP.

3. Touch R toe to the R side. Simultaneously swing arms to the R.

4. Return to SP.

E. Grapevine

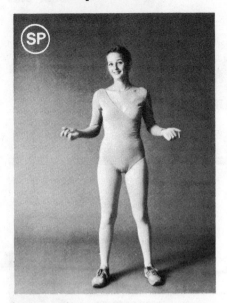

SP: Stand, arms bent at waist height.

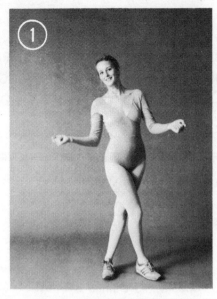

1. Bring R leg over and in front of L.

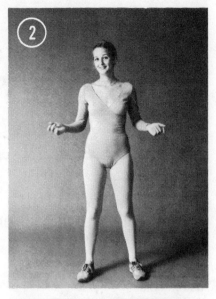

2. Bring L foot from behind R, and plant to the L.

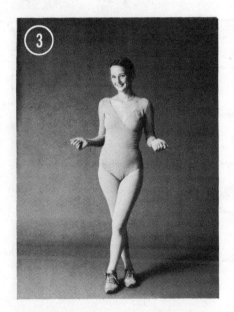

3. Bring R foot behind the L.

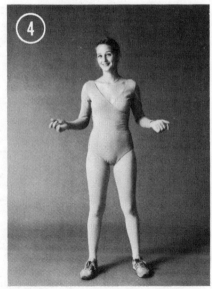

4. Move the L foot to the L.

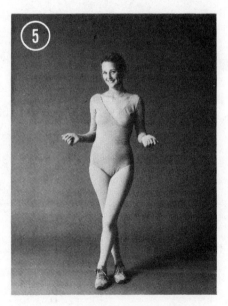

5. Do twice (8 steps total to L, then reverse direction bringing L leg over and in front of R).

7. Two Doors Down

low-intensity
time: 3:04

by Dolly Parton   RCA PB-11240

This easy routine (only three movements) combines a little country music and a little polka step to get your heart and legs moving to better figure fitness. Let Dolly help give you an hourglass figure for life.

MUSIC CUE	BEATS	ACTION	PICTURE CUE
instrumental	32	Double Hip Bumps	A
Two doors down . . .	32	Arrow Step	B
I think I'll . . .	32	Polka Step	C
Two doors down . . .	32	repeat Arrow Step	B
I can't believe . . .	32	repeat Polka Step	C
Two doors down . . .	32	repeat Arrow Step	B
Ha, Ha, Ho . . .	32	repeat Polka Step	C
Two doors down . . .	32	repeat Arrow Step	B
Two doors down . . .	32	repeat Polka Step	C

A. Double Hip Bumps

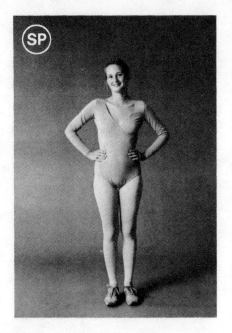

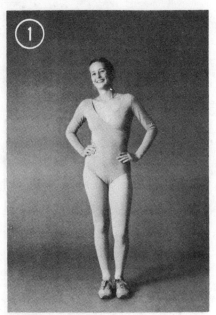

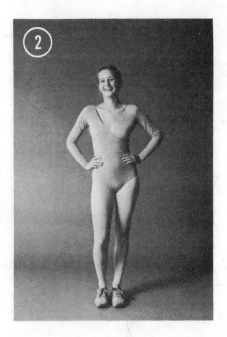

SP: Stand, hands on hips.

1. Rock R hip to R twice.

When rocking to R, R leg is straight and L leg is bent slightly at knee.

2. Rock L hip to L twice.

B. Arrow Step

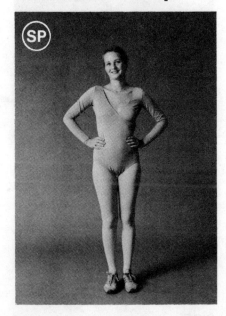

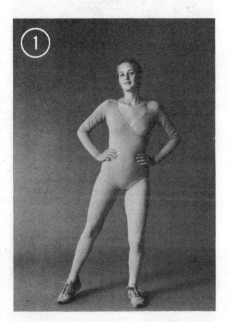

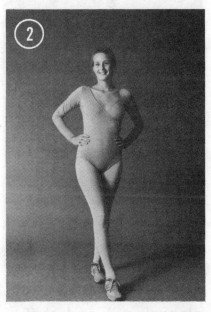

SP: Stand, hands on hips.

1. Touch R toe about 12" to R.

2. Touch R toe in front of L toe.

B. Arrow Step (Continued)

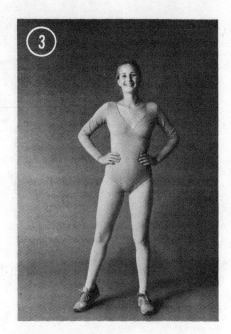

3. Repeat Step #1.

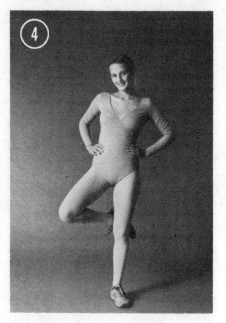

4. Bend R leg and touch R toe against and behind L knee.

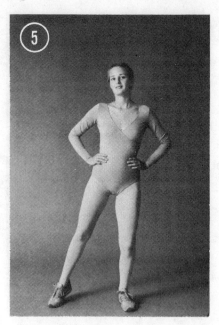

5. Repeat Step #1.

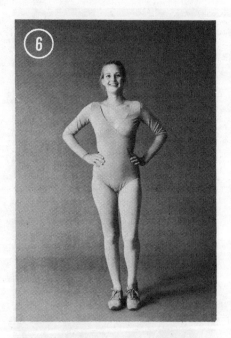

6. Bring R leg back alongside L and shift weight to R foot.

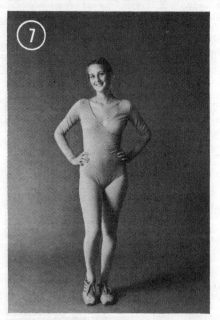

7. Walk forward with L and then R foot.

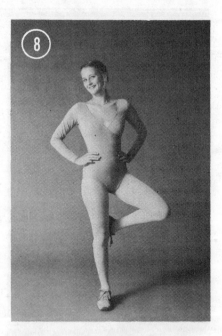

8. Repeat pattern on L side.

C. Polka Step

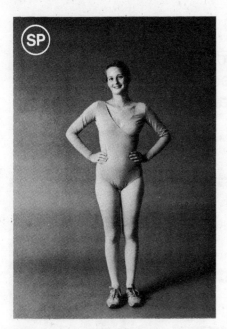

SP: Stand, hands on hips.

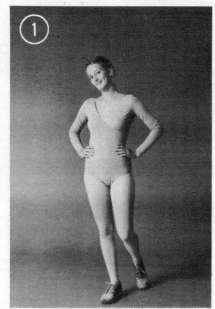

1. Put R foot forward and then put L foot alongside or behind R heel.

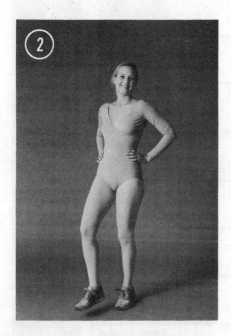

2. Step forward with R foot. Wait one beat.

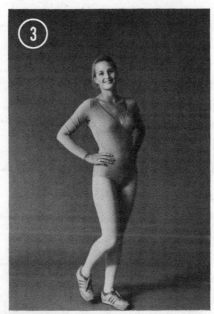

3. Repeat on L foot.

8. I'll Get Over You

by Crystal Gayle   United Artists US-XW1146

Here is a country and western tune that holds good $\frac{4}{4}$ time. This low-intensity exercise routine should be well tolerated by almost anyone regardless of their fitness level. If you are very fit and want a more strenuous workout from this routine, raise your legs higher as you walk or move.

MUSIC CUE	BEATS	ACTION	PICTURE CUE
instrumental	12	Shoulder Roll	A
One thing 'bout . . .	32	The Shovel	B
I'll find me . . .	16	Backwards Tilt	C
When I do . . .	16	Touch Behind	D
I'll get over . . .	8	Moving Arms Side	E
I'll get through . . .	8	Moving Arms Front	F
I'll be good . . .	8	Moving Arm Extensions	G
. . . I get over . . .	12	Moving Finger Snaps	H
From now on . . .	32	repeat The Shovel	B
Sometimes think I . . .	16	repeat Backwards Tilt	C
But I know . . .	16	repeat Touch Behind	D
I'll get over . . .	8	repeat Moving Arms Side	E

MUSIC CUE	BEATS	ACTION	PICTURE CUE

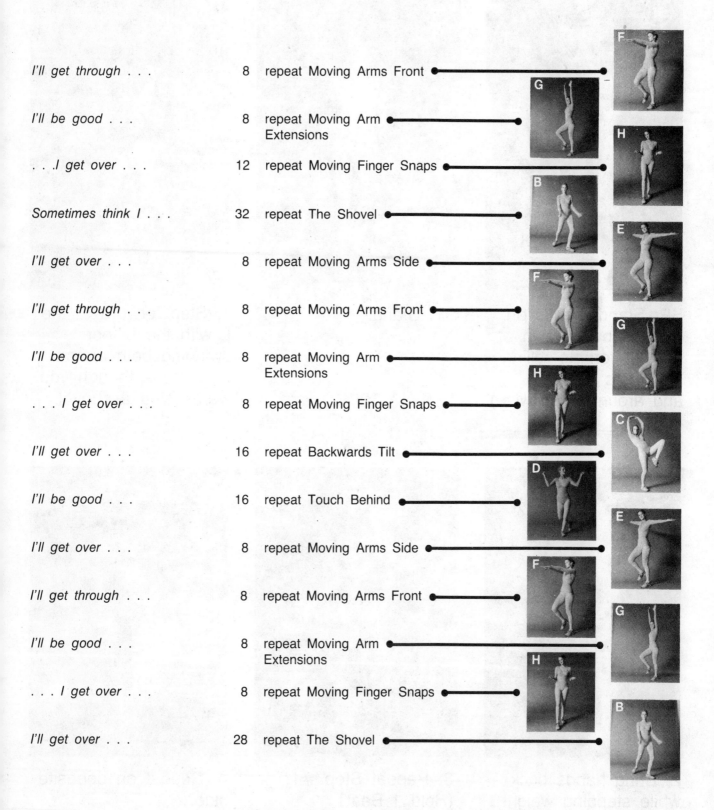

MUSIC CUE	BEATS	ACTION
I'll get through . . .	8	repeat Moving Arms Front
I'll be good . . .	8	repeat Moving Arm Extensions
. . .I get over . . .	12	repeat Moving Finger Snaps
Sometimes think I . . .	32	repeat The Shovel
I'll get over . . .	8	repeat Moving Arms Side
I'll get through . . .	8	repeat Moving Arms Front
I'll be good . . .	8	repeat Moving Arm Extensions
. . . I get over . . .	8	repeat Moving Finger Snaps
I'll get over . . .	16	repeat Backwards Tilt
I'll be good . . .	16	repeat Touch Behind
I'll get over . . .	8	repeat Moving Arms Side
I'll get through . . .	8	repeat Moving Arms Front
I'll be good . . .	8	repeat Moving Arm Extensions
. . . I get over . . .	8	repeat Moving Finger Snaps
I'll get over . . .	28	repeat The Shovel

A. Shoulder Roll

B. The Shovel

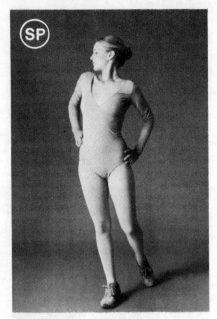

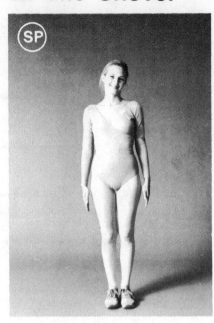

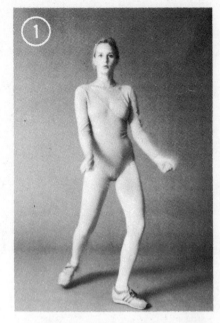

SP: Stand, hands on hips, elbows drawn back. Alternate rolling shoulders up, back, and around (clockwise).

SP: Stand.

1. Step forward to the L with the L foot, swinging both arms forward as though you were using a shovel.

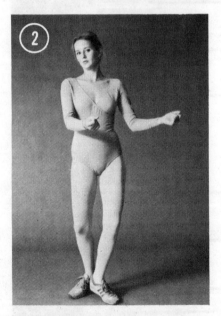

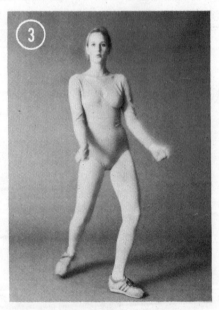

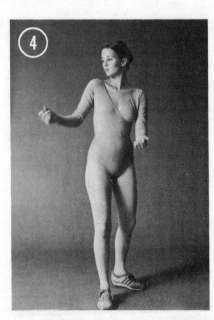

2. Bring hands back while stepping weight on R behind L.

3. Repeat Step #1. (Hold 1 Beat)

4. Repeat on opposite side.

C. Backwards Tilt

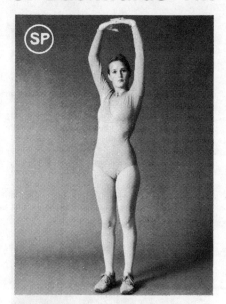 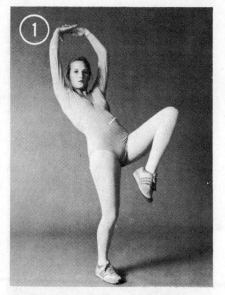 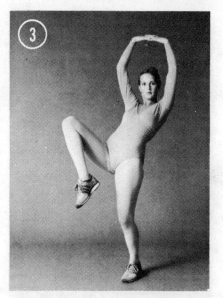

SP: Stand with arms extended overhead, hands clasped.

1. Raise the L knee while leaning backwards.
2. Drop leg, but keep arms extended.

3. Do Step #1 with the R leg.
4. Repeat Step #2.

D. Touch Behind

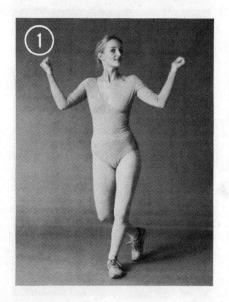 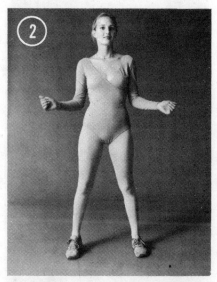 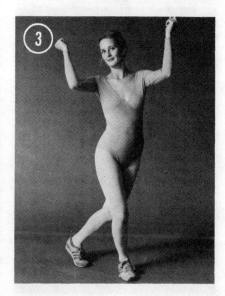

SP: Stand.
1. Touch R toes behind L leg. Raise arms and snap fingers.

2. Bring R foot even with L foot about shoulder width apart.

3. Repeat on other side.

E. Moving Arms Side

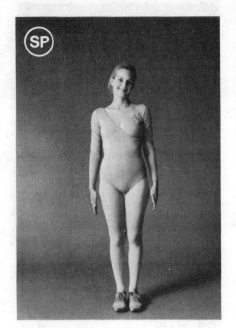

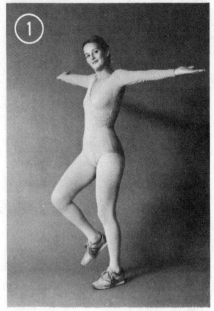

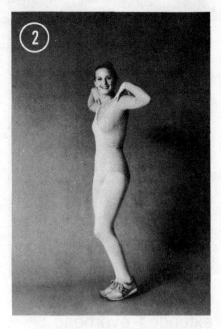

SP: Stand.

1. Walk in place, and extend the arms out to the sides.

2. Continue walking, and bring arms in so hands touch shoulders.

F. Moving Arms Front

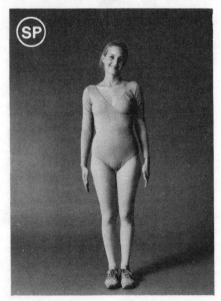

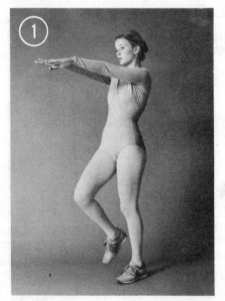

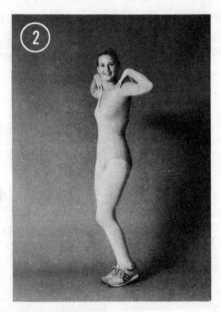

SP: Stand.

1. Walk in place, and extend the arms forward in front of the body.

2. Continue walking, and bring arms in so hands touch shoulders.

G. Moving Arm Extensions

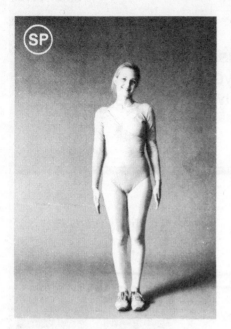 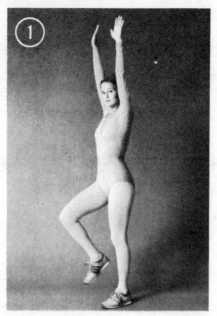 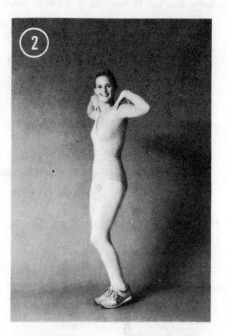

SP: Stand.

1. Walk in place, and extend the arms above the head.

2. Continue walking, and bring arms in so hands touch shoulders.

H. Moving Finger Snaps

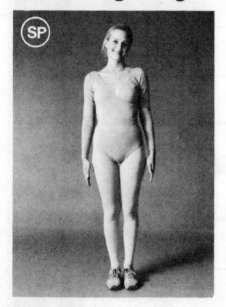 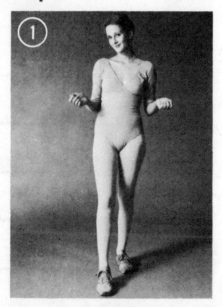 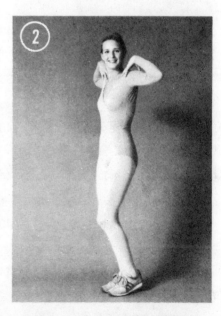

SP: Stand.

1. While walking in place with arms at sides, snap fingers.

2. Continue walking, and bring arms up so hands touch shoulders.

9. Love Will Keep Us Together

**moderate-intensity
time: 3:15**

by The Captain & Tennile   A&M 8590

Most of these steps can be learned quickly and easily. Some of the movements are vigorous, others a little less so. If you are very fit make your moves dramatic and vigorous. Don't pause between exercises and dance moves.

MUSIC CUE	BEATS	ACTION	PICTURE CUE
instrumental	16	¼ Knee Bends	A
Love, love will . . .	40	Arm Flings	B
. . . stop 'cause I . . .	40	Kick-2-3 Switch	C
You, you belong . . .	40	repeat Arm Flings	B
. . . stop 'cause I . . .	40	repeat Kick-2-3 Switch	C
Young and beautiful . . .	36	Jumping Jacks	D
. . . will be there . . .	40	Body Twist	E
. . . stop 'cause I . . .	44	repeat Kick-2-3 Switch	C
. . . will. instrumental	40	Walking Shoulder Rolls	F
. . . stop 'cause I . . .	44	repeat Kick-2-3 Switch	C
. . . will. instrumental	56	repeat Walking Shoulder Rolls	F

A. ¼ Knee Bends

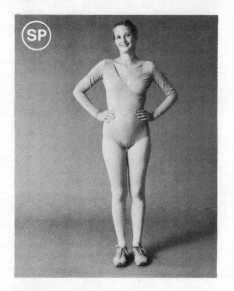 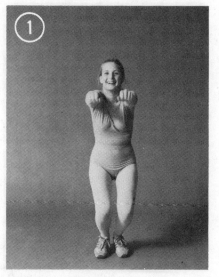 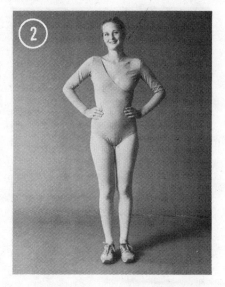

SP: Stand, hands on hips.

1. Bend the knees. Simultaneously extend arms in front of you. Keep arms parallel to the floor.

2. Return to SP.

B. Arm Flings

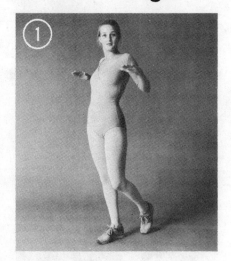 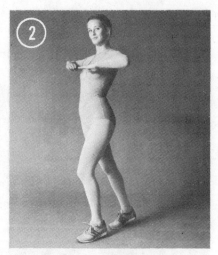 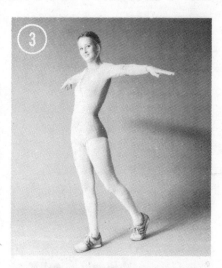

SP: Walk.

1. Swing both elbows backward.

2. Draw elbows forward.

3. Extend the arms at the elbows, and fling arms backward.

4. Repeat Step #2.

C. Kick-2-3 Switch

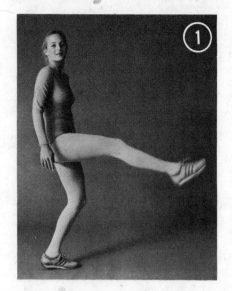

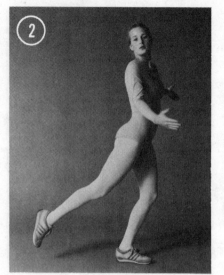

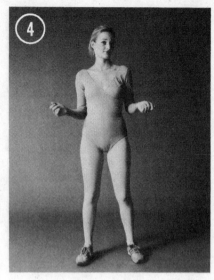

SP: Stand, arms at sides, elbows bent.

1. Swing R leg forward.

2. Swing R leg backward.

3. Swing R leg forward again.

4. Return to SP.

5. Repeat on L side.

D. Jumping Jacks

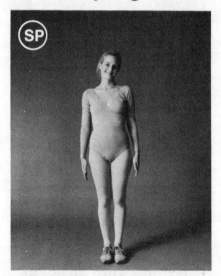

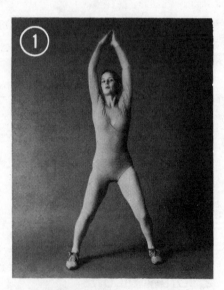

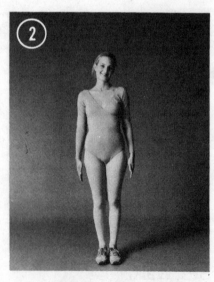

SP: Stand, feet together, arms at sides.

1. Jump and spread legs apart. Simultaneously swing arms upward and above head.

2. Jump back to SP with feet together. Lower arms to side.

E. Body Twist

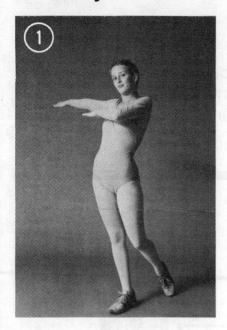

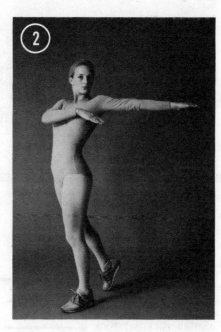

SP: Walk.

1. Step with R foot, swing R arm out to the side (keep parallel to floor). Draw L arm across the chest. Keep L arm also parallel to floor. Swing R arm back as far as possible.

2. Repeat Step #1 stepping on L foot, swinging L arm out to side, and drawing R arm across chest.

F. Walking Shoulder Rolls

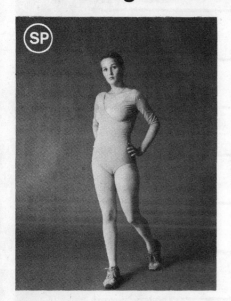

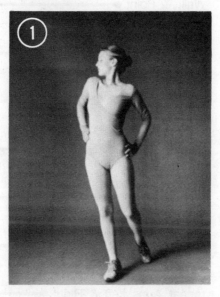

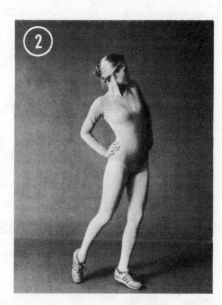

SP: Walk, hands on waist.

1. Roll the R shoulder up, around, and down (clockwise). Look over rolling shoulder.

2. Repeat with L shoulder.

10. I Will Survive

moderate-intensity
time: 3:15

by Gloria Gaynor Polydor 14508

A moderate workout, this routine starts slowly and builds. After the first few measures you start hopping as you move into more vigorous exercise. But, don't worry. We have paced this routine so you will survive and not fall apart. Keep moving.

MUSIC CUE	BEATS	ACTION	PICTURE CUE
First I was . . .	32	Leg Brush	A
. . . back from outer . . .	16	Small Kick/Big Kick	B
. . . changed that stupid . . .	16	Arms Left & Right	C
. . . go, walk out . . .	64	Fencing Hops	D
. . . hey.	32	Walk & Point	E
. . . all the strength . . .	32	repeat Leg Brush	A
. . . me, somebody new . . .	16	repeat Small Kick/Big Kick	B
. . . felt like droppin' . . .	16	repeat Arms Left & Right	C
. . . go. walk out . . .	64	repeat Fencing Hops	D
. . . I, I will . . .	32	(slows but keep jogging)	B
. . . go, walk out . . .	16	repeat Small Kick/Big Kick	C
Weren't you the . . .	16	repeat Arms Left & Right	A
. . . I, I will . . .	32	repeat Leg Brush	

CONSUMER GUIDE®

A. Leg Brush

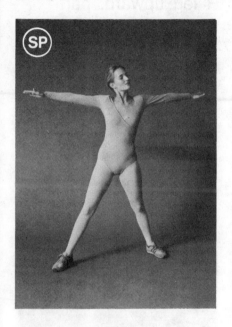

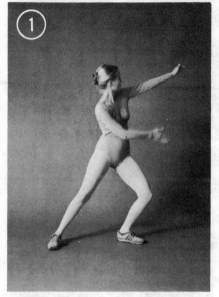

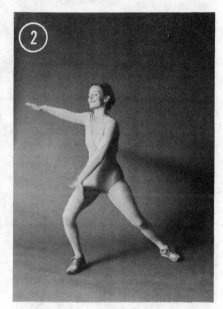

SP: Stand, feet wider than shoulder-width apart, toes pointed outward, arms stretched sideward and parallel to the floor.

1. Bend L knee to the L, knee pointing outward. Simultaneously sweep R arm down as a pendulum. Brush against inside of L thigh and swing arm upward and around to starting position.

2. Repeat, bending R knee and swinging L arm.

B. Small Kick/Big Kick

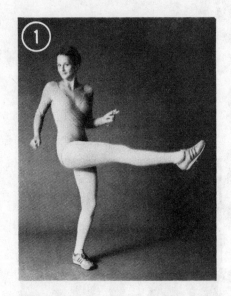

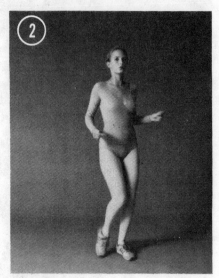

SP: Stand, hands on waist or at sides.

1. On beat 1, kick the R leg upward, part way.

2. On beat 2, lower R leg to floor.

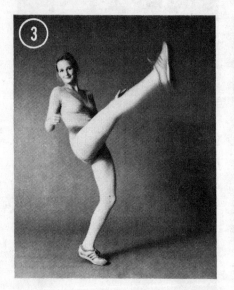

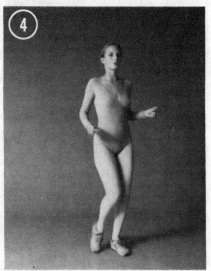

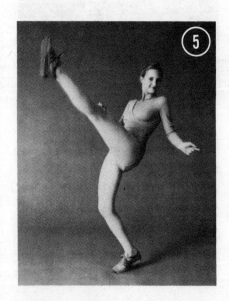

3. On beat 3, kick the R leg higher than in the first kick.

4. On beat 4, lower leg to floor.

5. Repeat on L side. This sequence works well while hopping.

C. Arms Left & Right

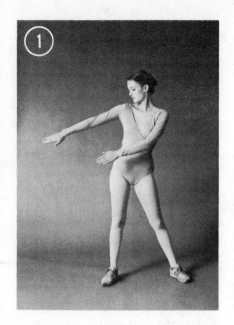

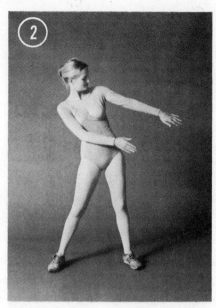

SP: Stand, feet slightly more than shoulder-width apart, arms at sides.

1. Swing the arms in front of the body to the R. Turn head and rock hips in direction of arms.

2. Swing arms back, and repeat to the L side.

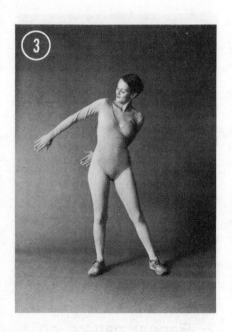

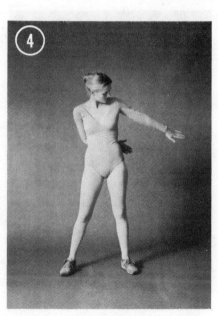

3. Swing the arms behind the body and to the R. Turn head and rock hips in direction of arms.

4. Swing arms back and repeat to the L side.

D. Fencing Hops

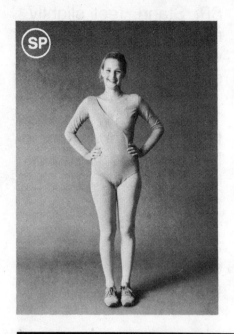

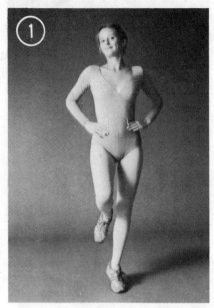

SP: Stand, hands on hips.

1. Hop on one foot, keeping the other knee bent.
Perform as follows: Hop 8 times on R, 8 times on L, 4 times on R, 4 times on L, 2 times on R, and 2 times on L. Then jog 4 beats at end.

E. Walk & Point

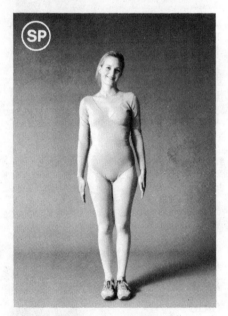

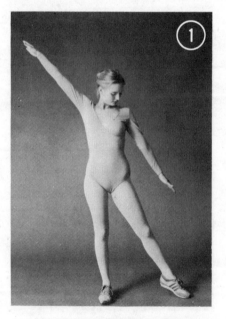

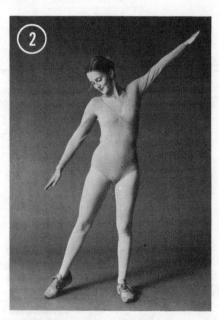

SP: Stand.

1. Walk 3 steps. On the 4th step point L foot to side. Extend R arm up and to the right, and extend L arm parallel to L leg.

2. Repeat pattern on other side.

11. Love Pollution

by Q   Epic 8-50335

This happy routine takes you from a stand-up position down to the floor and back again. One cautionary note: Learn this routine well so you can keep moving and work your cardiovascular system and burn more calories. Here is a routine that is designed to move your "you know what."

MUSIC CUE	BEATS	ACTION	PICTURE CUE
instrumental	8	Walk in Place	A
instrumental	8	Butterfly Hops	B
. . . love pollution all . . .	16	Kick Step	A
Particles of happiness . . .	20	repeat Butterfly Hops (Do 2½ times)	C
Together we can . . .	4	Walk-Down	D
. . . give it a . . .	4	rollover	
Don't let no . . .	16	4 Beat Sit-Up	E
. . . tell someone you . . .	4	rollover	
Before it is . . .	4	Walk-Up	F
. . . love pollution all . . .	16	Box Step	G
Particles of happiness . . .	8	Amos Moses-Part I	H
Pollute the air . . .	12	Amos Moses-Part II	A
. . . please don't love . . .	32	repeat Butterfly Hops	B
. . . love pollution all . . .	16	repeat Kick Step	

MUSIC CUE	BEATS	ACTION	PICTURE CUE
Particles of happiness . . .	20	repeat Butterfly Hops (Do 2½ times)	A
. . . love pollution all . . .	32	repeat Walk-Down;	C
		rollover; 4 Beat Sit-Up;	D
		rollover; Walk-Up	E
We need love . . .	36	repeat Box Step	F
. . . love pollution all . . .	36	repeat Butterfly Hops (Do 4½ times)	A
. . . love pollution all . . .	16	repeat Kick Step	B
Particles of happiness . . .	20	repeat Butterfly Hops (Do 2½ times)	A
. . . love pollution all . . .	36	repeat Walk-Down;	C
		rollover; 4 Beat Sit-Up;	D
		rollover; Walk-Up	E

A. Butterfly Hops

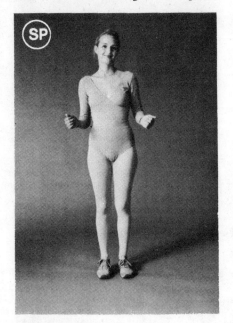

SP: Stand.

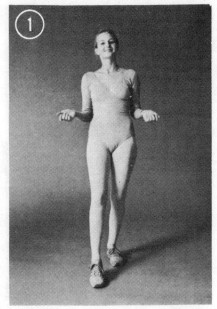

1. Touch R toe about 6" to front.

2. Bring it back to place.

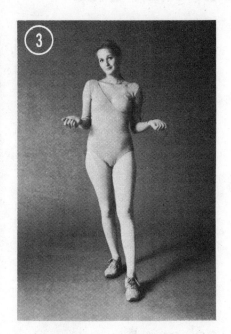

3. Touch L toe to front.

4. Bring it back to place.

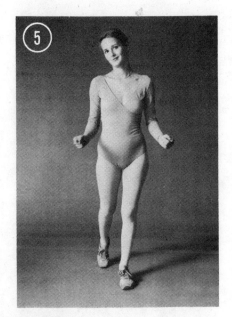

5. Touch R toe behind about 6".

6. Bring it back to place.

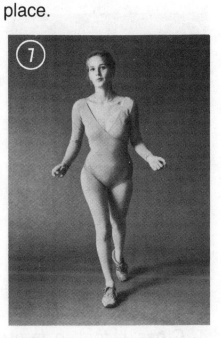

7. Touch L toe behind about 6".

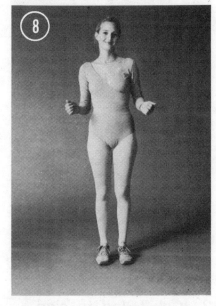

8. Bring it back to place. This sequence can all be done with hopping steps.

B. Kick Step

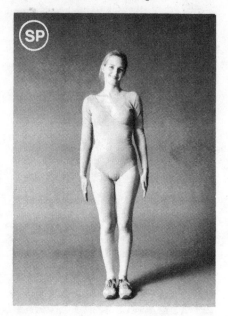

SP: Stand.

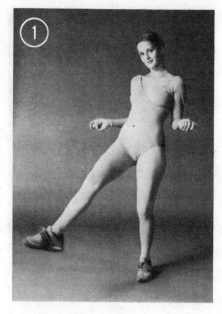

1. Kick R leg to R side about 12" from floor.

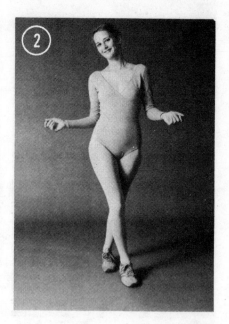

2. Cross R foot in front of L foot, and shift weight to R foot.

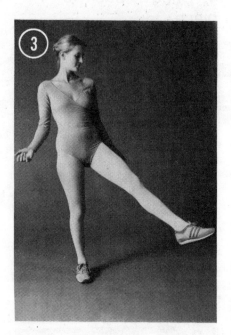

3. Kick L leg to side.

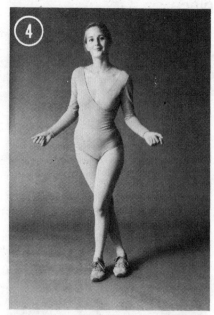

4. Cross L foot in front of R foot, and shift weight to L foot.

C. Walk-Down

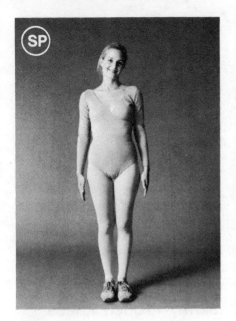

SP: Stand.

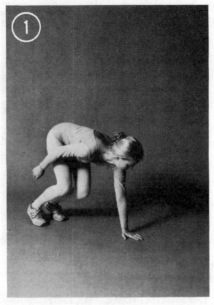

1. Lean forward, put L hand on floor. Place weight on L hand.

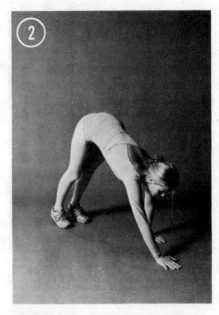

2. Place R hand on floor 8-12" in front of L hand.

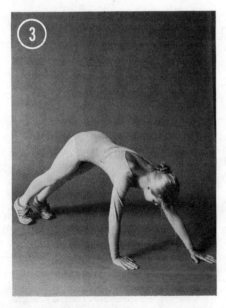

3. Then place L hand on floor ahead of R.

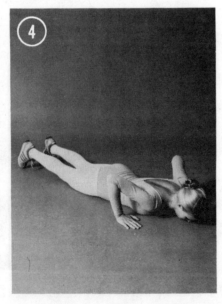

4. Drop body to floor into a push-up position.

D. rollover; 4 Beat Sit-Up

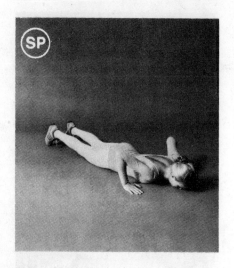

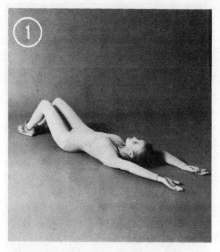

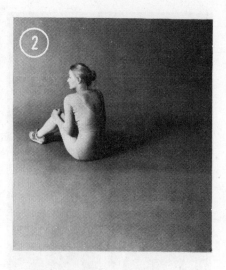

SP: Push-up position.

1. From push-up position take 4 beats to roll over on back. When on back, knees are to be bent, feet on floor, and arms extended above head.

2. Start to sit up slowly. Touch knees with hands.

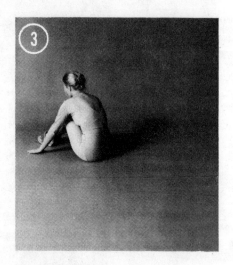

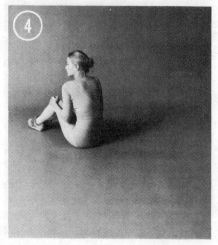

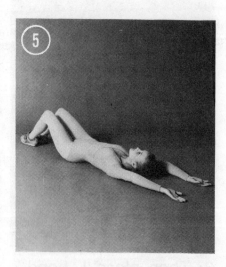

3. Touch floor with hands.

4. Touch hands to knees.

5. Slowly start to return to floor. (Sit-Up and return to floor take 4 beats.)

E. rollover; Walk-Up

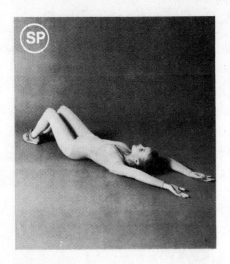

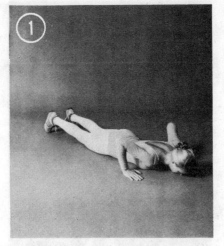

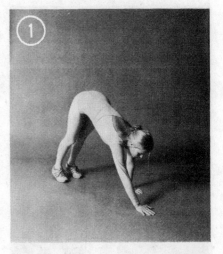

SP: Lie on back, knees bent; feet on floor.

1. Roll over onto stomach, taking 4 beats. Reverse Walk Down. That is, push up with hands and walk

hands backward toward feet until in standing position. Take 4 beats to walk up into upright position.

F. Box Step

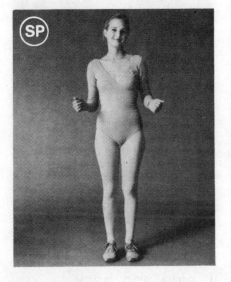

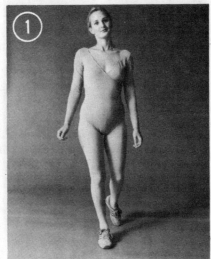

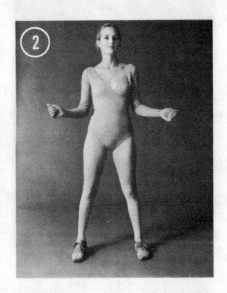

SP: Stand.

1. Step forward with R foot. Shift weight to R foot.

2. Step L foot forward, bringing L foot about 12" from R.

F. Box Step (Continued)

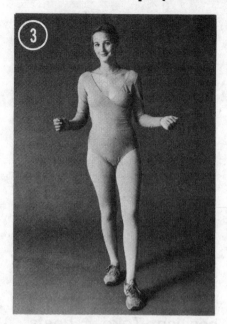

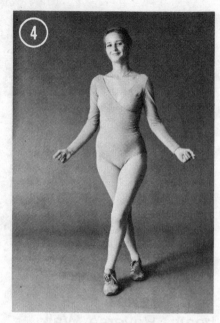

3. Step back with R foot, so that R foot is to the R of and about 6'' behind L foot.

4. Cross L foot over R foot.

G. Amos Moses-Part I

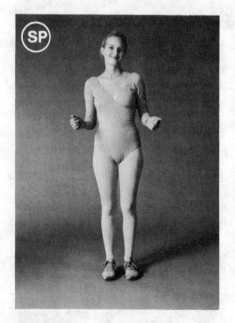

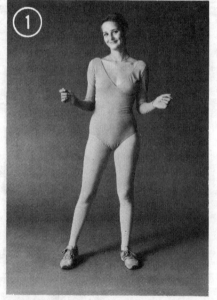

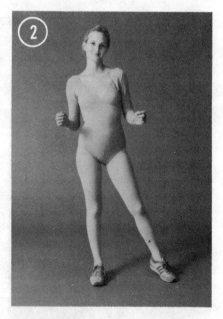

SP: Stand.

1. Touch R foot to R side (about 6-12'' from L foot) and bring back in place. Repeat. (Takes 4 Beats)

2. Now touch L foot to L side and back. Repeat.

H. Amos Moses-Part II

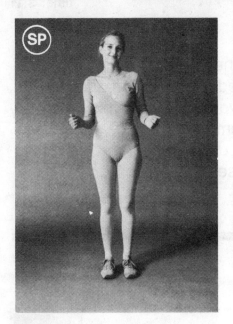

SP: Stand.

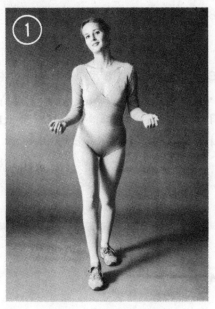

1. Step forward with R foot.

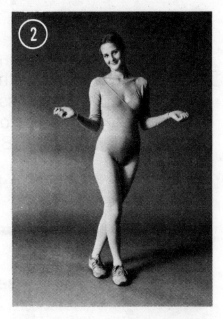

2. Cross L foot behind R foot, putting weight on L foot.

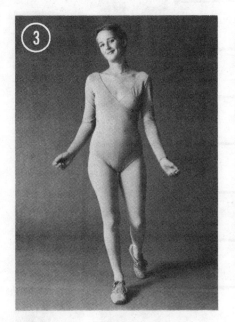

3. Step forward again with R foot.

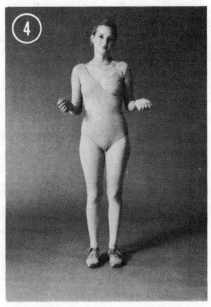

4. Bring L foot to the side of R foot.

12. Don't Stop

by Fleetwood Mac   Warner Bros. 8413

If a flatter middle is what you want, here's a routine that will help you realize that dream. All these exercises are designed to condition the muscles which crisscross your abdomen. At first, you may find this routine tires out your stomach muscles. It's one tummy-trimming exercise after another. But, soon you'll be able to do all of them nonstop. And when you can, you'll like what you see in the mirror. Remember: *Don't Stop!* Let the exercises flow.

MUSIC CUE	BEATS	ACTION	PICTURE CUE
instrumental	16	Up Oars	A
instrumental	16	Bicycle Pumps	B
If you wake . . .	32	Bent Knee Leg Raises	C
Don't stop thinking . . .	32	Side Bicycle Pumps	D
instrumental	16	Leg Shoot	E
Why not think . . .	16	Inverted Bicycle	F
If your life . . .	16	High Hips With Leg Raises	G
Don't stop thinking . . .	32	repeat Side Bicycle Pumps	D
instrumental	16	Single Arm and Leg Raises	H
instrumental	16	Mountain Climbers	I
instrumental	16	Knee Push-Ups	J

MUSIC CUE	BEATS	ACTION	PICTURE CUE
All I want . . .	16	repeat Mountain Climbers	
I know you . . .	16	repeat Single Arm and Leg Raises	
Don't stop thinking . . .	32	repeat Side Bicycle Pumps	
Don't stop thinking . . .	32	Underside Leg Raises	
Oooh . . . don't you . . .	16	repeat Bent Knee Leg Raises	
Oooh . . . don't you . . .	16	repeat Single Arm and Leg Raises	
Oooh . . . don't you . . .	24	repeat Bicycle Pumps	

A. Up Oars

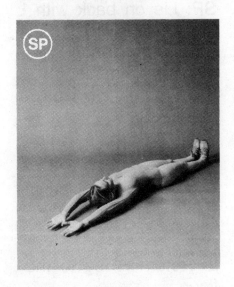

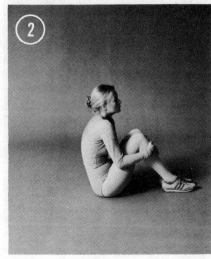

SP: Lie on back with arms overhead, legs extended.

1. Curl upper body off the floor, and simultaneously bend knees, sliding feet toward buttocks. Don't arch back.

2. Grasp hands around shins.

3. Return to SP.

B. Bicycle Pumps

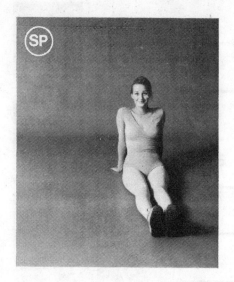 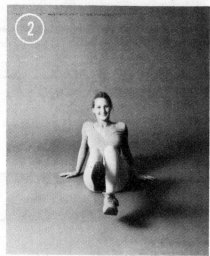

SP: Sit with legs extended and hands on floor beside hips.

1. Raise legs off the floor, and lean upper body back slightly.

2. Move legs as though riding a bicycle. Keep the back slightly rounded.

C. Bent Knee Leg Raises

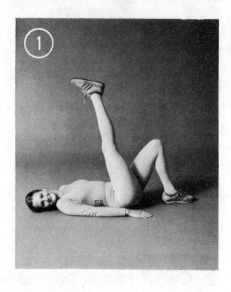 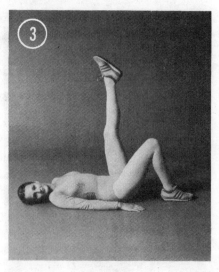

SP: Lie on back with L knee bent and L foot on floor. Extend R leg along the floor and place hands on hips or at sides.

1. Raise R leg, keeping small of back against floor.

2. Return R leg to the floor.

3. Raise R leg for half the beats. Then raise L leg for half the beats.

D. Side Bicycle Pumps

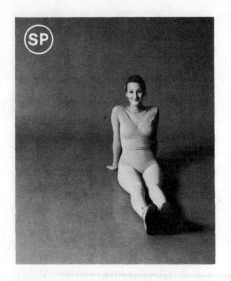

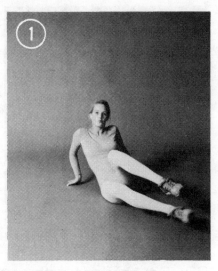

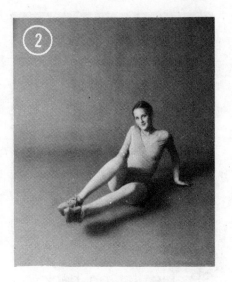

SP: Sit with legs extended and hands on floor behind hips. Raise legs off the floor and lean upper body back slightly. Shift weight to the R buttock.

1. Move legs as though riding a bicycle.

2. Do half the beats on R buttock and half the beats on L buttock.

E. Leg Shoot

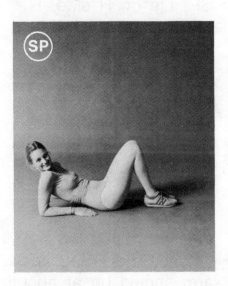

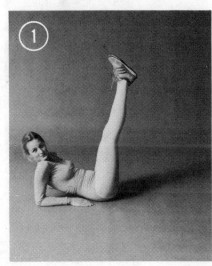

SP: Sit on the floor, knees bent. Lean back, place weight on forearms.

1. Quickly extend legs upward at an 80° or 90° angle.

2. Bend knees, and tap the floor with toes.

F. Inverted Bicycle   G. High Hips With Leg Raises

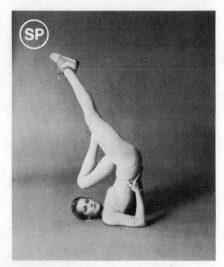

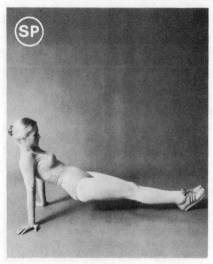

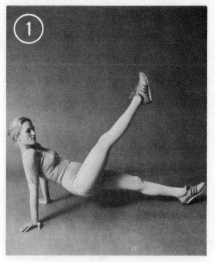

SP: Lie flat on back and raise both legs into air. Place hands on small of back for support. Place weight on shoulders. Pedal legs as though you were riding a bicycle.

SP: Sit on floor with legs extended. Keep hands on floor and behind hips. Raise hips off the floor about 5".

1. Alternately raise one leg to a 45° angle and then the other.

H. Single Arm And Leg Raises

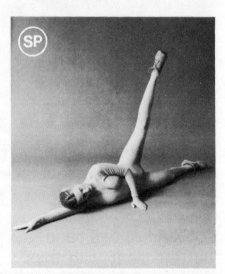

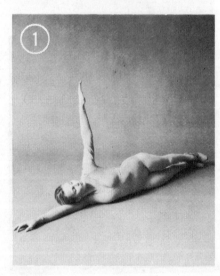

SP: Lie on R side, R arm extended above head (palm against floor). Head should be resting on extended arm. Raise L leg to at least a 45° angle.

1. Lower the L leg, and simultaneously raise the L arm. By the time the L leg touches the R leg, the arm should be at about a 90° angle.

H. Single Arm And Leg Raises (Continued)

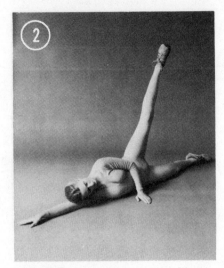

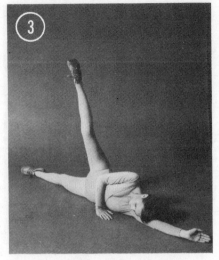

2. Return arm to starting position. Simultaneously raise leg.

3. Do half the beats lying on R side, then turn over and do half the beats lying on L side.

I. Mountain Climbers

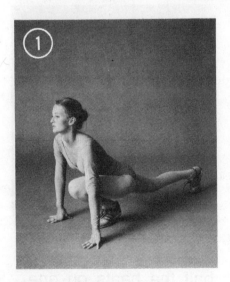

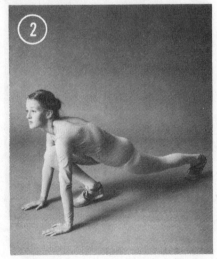

SP: Crouch, both hands on the floor, knees bent underneath the chest.

1. Extend R leg backward.

2. Reverse legs.

J. Knee Push-Ups

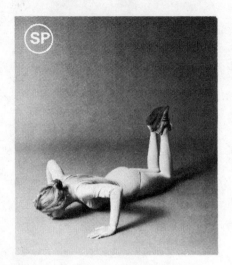

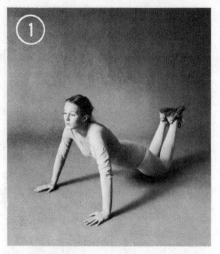

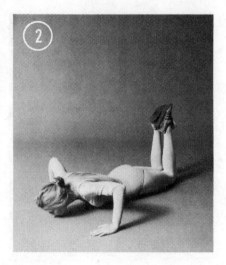

SP: Lie flat on stomach, legs together, knees bent. Hands palms down, beside shoulders.

1. Raise the torso and thighs until supported by hands and knees only.

2. Return to the SP.

K. Underside Leg Raises

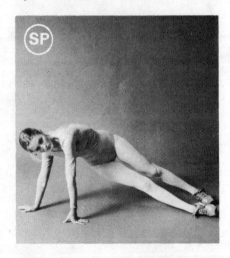

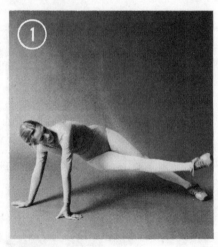

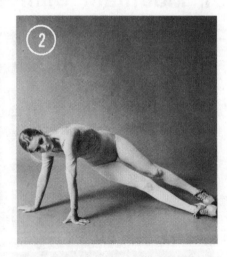

SP: Lie on R side. Place hands on floor. Push upper body off floor. Keep body rigid, so that your weight is supported entirely by feet and hands.

1. Raise bottom leg upward as high as possible.

2. Return to SP. Do half the beats on one side. Then roll over and do remaining beats on other side.

13. Back In The U.S.A.

by Linda Ronstadt   Asylum 45519

high-intensity
time: 3:02

Here's a high-intensity routine that will get your heart pumping and body hopping. This routine is to be done only by the very fit. If at any time you feel breathless, don't hop as high. Remember, keep moving fast enough to get your heartbeat up to its target rate.

MUSIC CUE	BEATS	ACTION	PICTURE CUE
instrumental	16	Swivel Hips	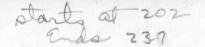
instrumental	32	Step Touch	
. . . well, oh, well, . . .	96	Popcorn Hops (do entire sequence twice)	
instrumental	48	repeat Step Touch	
Did I miss . . .	48	repeat Popcorn Hops (do once)	
instrumental	48	repeat Step Touch	
. . . high for a . . .	48	repeat Popcorn Hops (do once)	
I'm so glad . . .	48	repeat Swivel Hips	
We're so glad . . .	48	Opposite Knee Slaps	
We're so glad . . .	32	repeat Swivel Hips	
instrumental	16	repeat Opposite Knee Slaps	

A. Swivel Hips

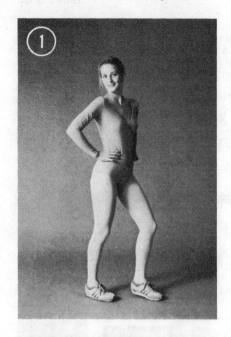 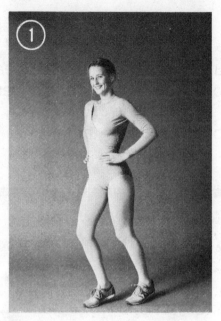

SP: Stand with hands on hips.

1. Pivot on the balls and heels of feet. Swing hips from R to L. Pivot 8 times in one direction and then reverse.

B. Step Touch

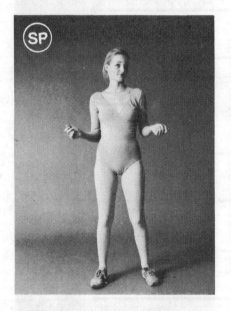 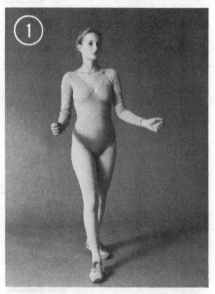 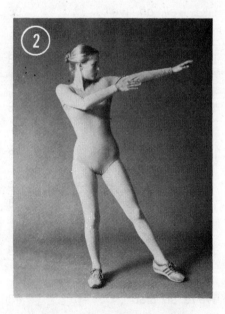

SP: Stand, arms at sides, elbows bent.

1. Step forward with R foot.

2. Shift weight to R foot, tap L toe to the side, and extend arms to the L.

3. Repeat on L side.

C. Popcorn Hops

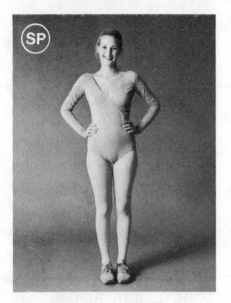

SP: Stand, both hands on hips.

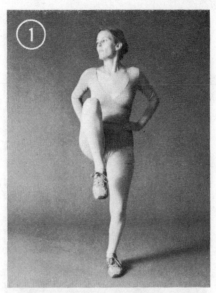

1. Hop 4 times on L foot, raising R knee. Return R foot to floor between hops each time. Repeat on opposite leg.

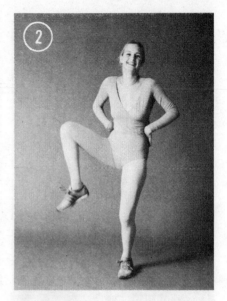

2. Hop on L foot, raising R knee to the side. Return R foot to floor between hops each time. Hop 4 times on the L; then hop 4 times on the R.

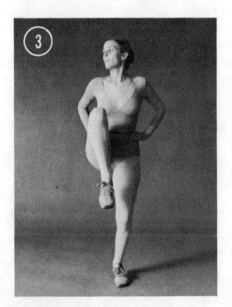

3. Hop 2 times on each foot, raising knee to the front.

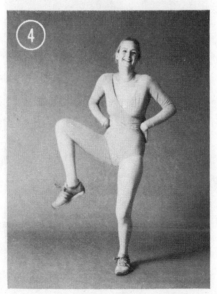

4. Hop once on each foot, raising knee to the side.

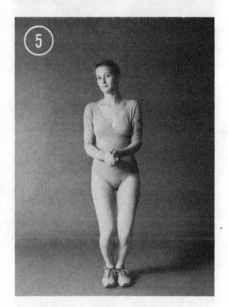

5. Clap and hop simultaneously—wait 1 beat. Repeat clap/hop/wait sequence.

D. Opposite Knee Slaps

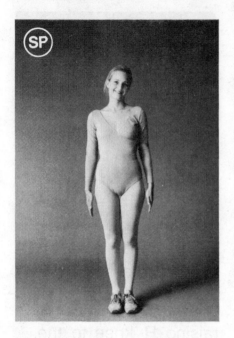

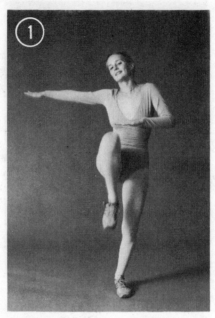

SP: Stand with arms at sides.

1. Hop on the L foot and raise R knee to waist height. Extend R arm to the side and bring L arm across body. Tap L hand to top of R knee.

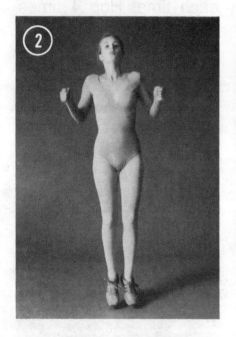

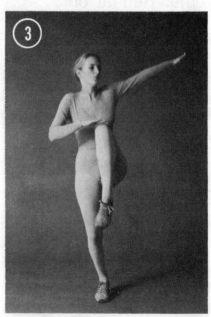

2. Bring L leg down, hop on both feet.

3. Repeat on other side.

14. Stumblin' In

by Suzi Quatro & Chris Norman   RSO 917

high-intensity
time: 3:28

A high-intensity routine with a rock beat, that's what "Stumblin' In" is. This routine works your legs, arms, and cardiovascular system. Move and get your heart and lungs really working.

MUSIC CUE	BEATS	ACTION	PICTURE CUE
. . . alive, and so . . .	32	Running Double Arm Pumps	A
. . . flame burnin' within . . .	32	Skier's Exercise	B
. . . go, whatever you . . .	32	Side Stretch—¼-Knee Bend	C
. . . you, whatever you . . .	32	Knee Hop Side Touch	D
. . . takes, baby I'll . . .	16	Side Kicks	E
. . . alive, and so . . .	32	repeat Running Double Arm Pumps	A
. . . flame burnin' within . . .	32	repeat Skier's Exercise	B
instrumental	32	Hops	F
. . . young and I . . .	32	repeat Side Stretch—¼-Knee Bend	C
. . . one. Oh, why . . .	32	repeat Knee Hop Side Touch	D
. . . need, baby you . . .	16	repeat Side Kicks	E

MUSIC CUE	BEATS	ACTION	PICTURE CUE

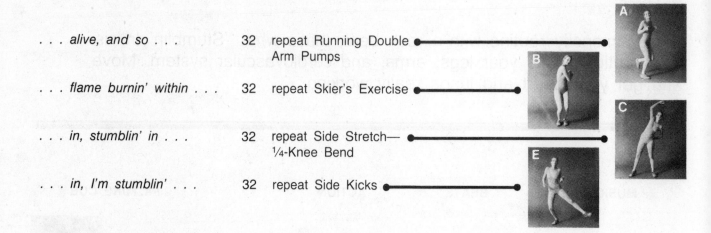

. . . alive, and so . . . — 32 — repeat Running Double Arm Pumps

. . . flame burnin' within . . . — 32 — repeat Skier's Exercise

. . . in, stumblin' in . . . — 32 — repeat Side Stretch—¼-Knee Bend

. . . in, I'm stumblin' . . . — 32 — repeat Side Kicks

A. Running Double Arm Pumps

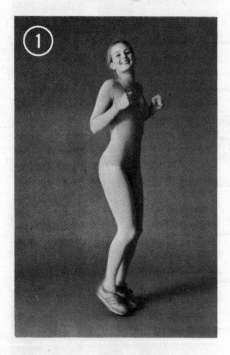

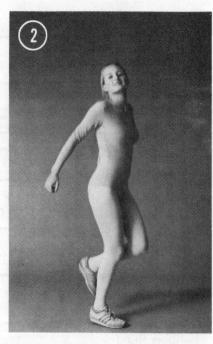

SP: Stand. Keep arms in close to body, fists clenched.

1. Run in place, pumping elbows backwards twice. (Takes 2 Beats)

2. Then swing arms forward slightly, down, and behind back. Return to SP. (Takes 2 Beats)

B. Skier's Exercise

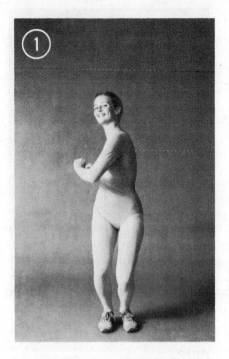

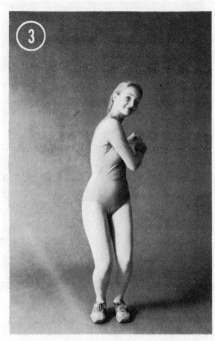

SP: Stand, feet together.

1. Do a ¼-knee bend. As you do, move both arms to the R as though you were using ski poles on that side.

2. Return to the SP.

3. Do a ¼-knee bend and move both arms to the L.

Note: Arms actually describe Figure 8's across the body from R to L.

C. Side Stretch—¼-Knee Bend

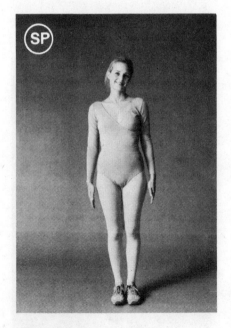

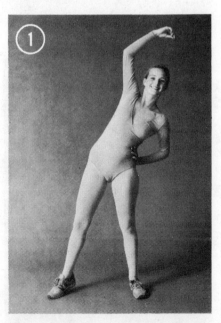

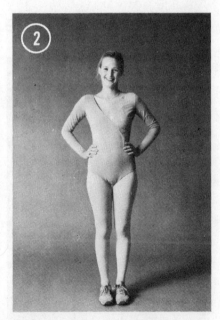

SP: Stand, feet together.

1. Extend R arm above the head, L hand on hip. Bend toward the L. (Takes 1 Beat)

2. Return to full upright position, hands on hips. (Takes 1 Beat)

C. Side Stretch—¼-Knee Bend (Continued)

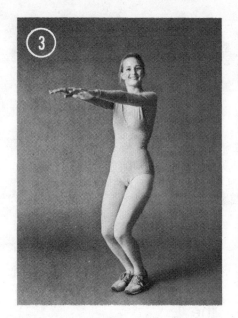

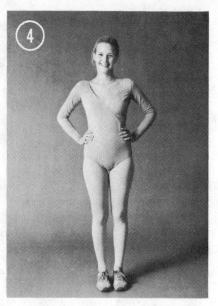

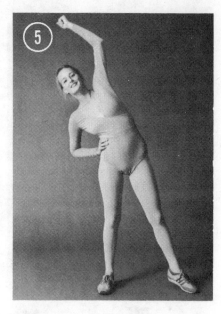

3. Do a ¼-knee bend and extend arms forward and parallel to floor. (Takes 1 Beat)

4. Return to full upright position, hands on hips. (Takes 1 Beat)

5. Repeat on other side.

D. Knee Hop Side Touch

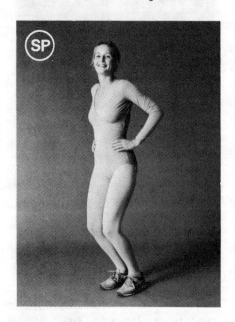

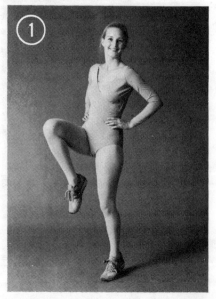

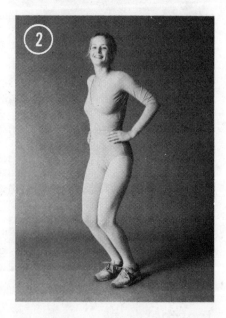

SP: Stand.

1. Hop on L foot, bring R knee up. (Takes 1 Beat)

2. Return to SP. (Takes 1 Beat)

D. Knee Hop Side Touch (Continued)

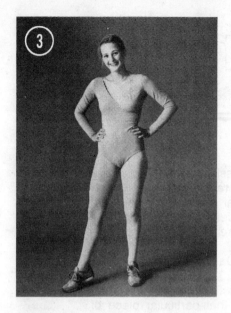

3. Then tap R foot to side. Return. (Takes 2 Beats)

4. Repeat on other side.

E. Side Kicks

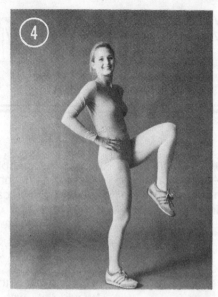

SP: Stand.

1. Alternately kick your L leg and then your R leg to the side.

F. Hops

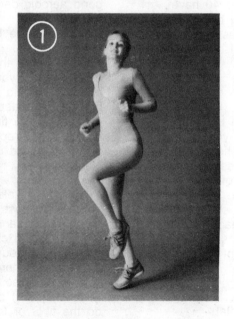

SP: Stand.

1. Hop lightly on R foot for 8 beats. When hopping, hold opposite leg up, knee bent.

2. Repeat on L side.

Doing Your Own Thing

By now you know there is nothing magical about putting together aerobic dance routines. You can make your own, and you may have already tried. Here are some guidelines.

Selecting the Music

Any time you listen to the radio, and find yourself tapping your foot or wanting to move, write down the name of the record.

Visit a record store and try to listen to as many musical selections as possible. If a particular number has good rhythm and you feel the urge to move you should consider buying it to develop your own aerobic routine. Most country music and the records that make it to the Top 40 have strong, consistent beats. When you begin, shy away from blues and jazz selections. For starters pick records that have lyrics. Vocal cues make it much easier to follow a routine.

Analyzing the Music

Most popular music can be broken down into segments of eight beats. Listen to your selection for its natural breakdown; you will hear recurring musical passages or series of passages, usually in segments of eight (or multiples of eight) beats. The selection will probably have an instrumental introduction, followed by either the chorus (theme), or the verse. Count the beats in each of these segments. Remember that musicians sometimes add interludes, making one segment 20 beats, instead of 16. Here is an example:

no. of beats	segment
8	instrumental
8	
4	
8	chorus
8	
8	
8	
8	verse
8	
8	
8	

Whenever possible write down the first few words of the phrase in each segment. That will give you a vocal cue to help separate the segments and determine when to repeat and change the exercise.

Selecting the Dance Steps

As you listen to the music, think about what steps would "fit" with that particular piece of music—high kicks, jumping jacks, or slow rhythmic stretches. Try them to the various segments of the music. If they seem to work, include them. If not, put them aside for future reference. Once you have five to 10 steps that you think will make a good aerobic dance routine move to . . .

Combining the Music and the Steps

Here is where the fun begins. Look at the breakdown of your musical selection. Each natural break, usually a segment of 16 to 32 beats, can probably be fitted to one exercise step. So your next task is to fit the steps to the music. Do not do too many repetitions of a particular exercise unless you find it particularly exciting and stimulating.

Hint: First select an exercise that fits the chorus. It's best to make the chorus exercises the most exciting and dramatic. Repeat that exercise every time the chorus is repeated. That's what we tried to do throughout the book. It makes it easier for you to remember the various exercises.

Most exercise patterns are in multiples of two (jumping jacks) or four (1-2-3 Kick). It is best to do the two- or four-beat patterns in 16-beat segments. If you really like one movement, you could do it for 32 beats.

Practice your new routine. Work on making the transition between the exercises smooth and continuous.

Don't be a purist. Be willing to change your steps. If you find that the steps and music don't seem to fit when you put them into a sequence, be ready to substitute a new movement. If you later find another step that you would like to use in place of a current exercise—use it.